T0229048

New Advances in Wrist and Small Joint Arthroscopy

Guest Editor

DAVID J. SLUTSKY, MD

HAND CLINICS

www.hand.theclinics.com

August 2011 • Volume 27 • Number 3

SAUNDERS an imprint of ELSEVIER, Inc.

W.B. SAUNDERS COMPANY
A Division of Elsevier Inc.

1600 John F. Kennedy Blvd. • Suite 1800 • Philadelphia, Pennsylvania 19103

http://www.theclinics.com

HAND CLINICS Volume 27, Number 3
August 2011 ISSN 0749-0712, ISBN-13: 978-1-4557-1100-0

Editor: Debora Dellapena
Developmental Editor: Donald Mumford

Hand Clinics (ISSN 0749-0712) is published quarterly by Elsevier Inc., 360 Park Avenue South, New York, NY 10010-1710. Months of publication are February, May, August, and November. Business and Editorial Offices: 1600 John F. Kennedy Blvd., Ste. 1800, Philadelphia, PA 19103-2899. Customer Service Office: 3251 Riverport Lane, Maryland Heights, MO 63043. Periodicals postage paid at New York, NY and at additional mailing offices. Subscription price is $338.00 per year (domestic individuals), $540.00 per year (domestic institutions), $169.00 per year (domestic students/residents), $385.00 per year (Canadian individuals), $617.00 per year (Canadian institutions), $459.00 per year (international individuals), $617.00 per year (international institutions), and $223.00 per year (international and Canadian students/residents). Foreign air speed delivery is included in all *Clinics* subscription prices. All prices are subject to change without notice. **POSTMASTER:** Send address changes to *Hand Clinics*, Elsevier Health Sciences Division, Subscription Customer Service, 3251 Riverport Lane, Maryland Heights, MO 63043. Customer Service (orders, claims, online, change of address): Elsevier Health Sciences Division, Subscription Customer Service, 3251 Riverport Lane, Maryland Heights, MO 63043. Tel: 1-800-654-2452 (U.S. and Canada); 314-447-8871 (outside U.S. and Canada). Fax: 314-447-8029. E-mail: journalscustomerservice-usa@elsevier.com (for print support); journalsonlinesupport-usa@elsevier.com (for online support).

Reprints. For copies of 100 or more of articles in this publication, please contact the Commercial Reprints Department, Elsevier Inc., 360 Park Avenue South, New York, New York 10010-1710. Tel.: 212-633-3812; Fax: 212-462-1935; E-mail: reprints@elsevier.com.

Hand Clinics is covered in *MEDLINE/PubMed (Index Medicus), Current Contents/Clinical Medicine, EMBASE/Excerpta Medica,* and *ISI/BIOMED.*

Printed and bound by CPI Group (UK) Ltd, Croydon, CR0 4YY

Transferred to Digital Print 2011

Contributors

GUEST EDITOR

DAVID J. SLUTSKY, MD
Assistant Clinical Professor, Department of
Orthopedics, Harbor-University of California,
The Hand and Wrist Institute, Torrance,
California

AUTHORS

JOSHUA M. ABZUG, MD
Assistant Professor, Department of
Orthopaedic Surgery, University of Maryland
School of Medicine, Baltimore, Maryland

JULIE E. ADAMS, MD
Assistant Professor, Department of
Orthopaedic Surgery, University of Minnesota,
Minneapolis, Minnesota

LARS ADOLFSSON, MD
Associate Professor, Department of
Orthopaedic Surgery, Linköping University
Hospital, Linköping, Sweden

ANDREA ATZEI, MD
Hand Surgery and Rehabilitation Team,
Treviso; Consultant Hand Surgeon at
Policlinico "San Giorgio", Pordenone;
Associate Professor, Department Orthopaedic
Surgery, Azienda Ospedaliera-Universitaria,
Verona, Italy

ALEJANDRO BADIA, MD
Badia Hand to Shoulder Center, Miami, Florida

GREGORY I. BAIN, MBBS, FRACS, PhD
Associate Professor; Senior Visiting
Orthopaedic Surgeon, Modbury Hospital;
Department of Orthopaedic Surgery, University
of Adelaide; Royal Adelaide Hospital, Adelaide,
South Australia, Australia

STACEY H. BERNER, MD
Advanced Centers for Orthopaedic Surgery
and Sports Medicine, Owings Mills, Maryland

MICHAEL V. BIRMAN, MD
Post-doctoral Clinical Fellow, Department of
Orthopaedic Surgery, Columbia University
Medical Center, New York, New York

**ALEXANDER K.Y. CHOI, MBChB,
FRCS(Edinburgh), FRCSEd(Ortho),
FHKCOS, FHKAM(Orthopaedic Surgery)**
Senior Medical Officer, Department of
Orthopaedics and Traumatology, Tuen Mun
Hospital, Hong Kong SAR, China

**ESTHER C.S. CHOW, MBBS, MRCS(Edin),
MMSc, FRCSEd(Ortho)**
Resident Specialist, Department of
Orthopaedics and Traumatology, Prince of
Wales Hospital; Honorary Clinical Tutor,
Department of Orthopaedics and
Traumatology, Faculty of Medicine, The
Chinese University of Hong Kong, Hong Kong
SAR, China

**Y.Y. CHOW, MBBS, FRCS(Edin), FRACS,
FHKCOS, FHKAM(Orthopaedic Surgery)**
Clinical Associate Professor (Honorary),
Department of Orthopaedics and
Traumatology, Faculty of Medicine, The
Chinese University of Hong Kong; Chief of
Service, Department of Orthopaedics and
Traumatology, Tuen Mun Hospital, Hong Kong
SAR, China

TYSON K. COBB, MD
Director of Hand Surgery, Orthopaedic
Specialists, Davenport, Iowa

RANDALL W. CULP, MD
Professor of Orthopedic and Hand Surgery,
Thomas Jefferson University, The Philadelphia
Hand Center, King of Prussia, Pennsylvania

JONATHAN R. DANOFF, MD
Post-doctoral Residency Fellow and Harrison
L. McLaughlin Research Fellow, Department of
Orthopaedic Surgery, Columbia University
Medical Center, New York, New York

F. DARIN, MD
Istituto Codivilla Putti, Orthopedica, Cortina
d'Ampezzo, Italy

FRANCISCO DEL PIÑAL, MD, DrMed
Unit of Hand-Wrist and Plastic Surgery,
Hospital Mutua Montañesa, Instituto de Cirugía
Plástica y de la Mano, Santander, Spain

ADAM W. DURRANT, MBChB, FRACS
Hand and Upper Limb Fellow, Orthopaedic
Department, Modbury Hospital, Modbury,
South Australia, Australia

WILLIAM B. GEISSLER, MD
Professor and Chief, Division of Hand and
Upper Extremity Surgery; Chief, Arthroscopic
Surgery and Sports Medicine, Department of
Orthopaedic Surgery and Rehabilitation,
University of Mississippi Health Care, Jackson,
Mississippi

**P.C. HO, MBBS, FRCS(Edinburgh),
FHKCOS, FHKAM(Orthopaedic Surgery)**
Consultant, Department of Orthopaedics and
Traumatology, Prince of Wales Hospital,
Shatin, N.T., Hong Kong; Clinical Associate
Professor (Honorary), Department of
Orthopaedics and Traumatology, Faculty of
Medicine, The Chinese University of Hong
Kong, Hong Kong SAR, China

HIROYASU IKEGAMI, MD, PhD
Department of Orthopaedic Surgery, School of
Medicine, Keio University, Tokyo, Japan

JOHN W. KARL, MD, MPH
Post-doctoral Residency Fellow and Harrison
L. McLaughlin Research Fellow, Department of
Orthopaedic Surgery, Columbia University
Medical Center, New York, New York

RICCARDO LUCHETTI, MD
Rimini Hand Center; Consultant of Wrist
Pathology, Department Hand Surgery,
Clinic of Plastic and Reconstructive Surgery,
Multimedica Milano, Rimini, Italy

C. MATHOULIN, MD
Professor, Institut de la Main, Clinique
Jouvenet, Paris, France

TOSHIYASU NAKAMURA, MD, PhD
Department of Orthopaedic Surgery, School
of Medicine, Keio University, Tokyo, Japan

MASATO OKAZAKI, MD
Department of Orthopaedic Surgery, School
of Medicine, Keio University, Tokyo, Japan

A. LEE OSTERMAN, MD
Professor, Department of Orthopaedic
Surgery, The Philadelphia Hand Center,
Thomas Jefferson University Hospital,
Philadelphia; The Philadelphia Hand Center,
King of Prussia, Pennsylvania

MELVIN P. ROSENWASSER, MD
Robert E. Carroll Professor of Hand Surgery
and Director, Orthopaedic Hand and Trauma
Services, Department of Orthopaedic Surgery,
Columbia University College of Physicians and
Surgeons, New York, New York

DOUGLAS M. SAMMER, MD
Assistant Professor, Department of Plastic
Surgery, UT Southwestern Medical Center,
Dallas, Texas

KAZUKI SATO, MD, PhD
Department of Orthopaedic Surgery, School
of Medicine, Keio University, Tokyo, Japan

ALEXANDER Y. SHIN, MD
Consultant and Professor, Department of
Orthopedic Surgery, Mayo Clinic, Rochester,
Minnesota

DAVID J. SLUTSKY, MD
Assistant Clinical Professor, Department of
Orthopedics, Harbor-University of California,
The Hand and Wrist Institute, Torrance,
California

SCOTT P. STEINMANN, MD
Professor, Department of Orthopedic Surgery, Mayo Clinic, Rochester, Minnesota

YOSHIAKI TOYAMA, MD, PhD
Department of Orthopaedic Surgery, School of Medicine, Keio University, Tokyo, Japan

THOMAS TRUMBLE, MD
Bellevue Bone and Joint Physicians, Affiliate Physician Overlake Hospital Medical Center, Department of Orthopaedic Surgery, Bellevue, Washington

W.Y. CLARA WONG, MBChB, MRCS, FRCSEd (Orth), FHKAM (Orthopaedic Surgery), FHKCOS
Department of Orthopaedics and Traumatology, Prince of Wales Hospital, Shatin, N.T., Hong Kong

JEFFREY YAO, MD
Assistant Professor of Orthopaedic Surgery, Department of Orthopaedic Surgery, Robert A. Chase Hand and Upper Limb Center, Stanford University Medical Center, Redwood City, California

Contents

Injury to the triangular fibrocartilage complex (TFCC) is a major source of ulnar-sided wrist pain that results in disability with common activities of daily living involving forearm rotation, for which operative management is indicated if conservative management fails. Past results with open repairs have been successful, but recent surgical advances have allowed the development of arthroscopic management. This article describes and reviews an all-arthroscopic technique of repair of Palmer type IB TFCC injuries with FasT-Fix suture technology (Smith and Nephew, Andover, MA, USA), which is advantageous both biomechanically and in terms of decreasing risk of morbidity.

The triangular fibrocartilage complex (TFCC) is the key structure at the wrist that facilitates the rotation of the radius and the carpus on the distal ulnar. The radial or type 1D tears of the TFCC are uncommon, but they pose a major disruption of the articular contact between the carpus and the distal ulna. The tears can heal by arthroscopically repairing the TFCC back to the radius using sutures through bone tunnels. This procedure allows patients to return to their work and sports activities with significant recovery of strength and range of motion.

Anatomical and biomechanical studies have highlighted the importance of the deep attachment of the TFCC for maintaining stability of the distal radioulnar joint (DRUJ). The standard arthroscopic assessment of the TFCC does not allow one to definitively determine whether the deep fibers are indeed intact, and establishing the diagnosis of a foveal detachment remains an exacting challenge. DRUJ arthroscopy is useful to assess the foveal fibers in any patient with DRUJ instability and can aid in the surgical decision making.

During the last two decades, increased knowledge of functional anatomy and pathophysiology of the triangular fibrocartilage complex (TFCC) have contributed to a change in surgeons' perspective toward it. The earlier concept of the TFCC as the "hammock" structure of the ulnar carpus has updated to the "iceberg" concept, whereby the much larger "submerged" part represents the foveal insertions of the TFCC and functions as the stabilizer of the distal radioulnar joint and the ulnar carpus, thus lending it greater functional importance. This article presents an

remove as much effusion and inflammatory substrate as possible. In most cases, arthroscopic synovectomy is performed as an outpatient procedure. The technique has also been used for other diagnoses causing wrist arthritis, but very few results have been reported and the indications remain to be defined. In rheumatoid arthritis (RA), juvenile chronic arthritis (JCA), systemic lupus erythematosus (SLE), and post-infectious monoarthritis, a long period of increased comfort and improved function can be anticipated.

Due to an administrative error, the following article was inadvertently omitted from this issue: "Arthroscopic Dorsal Capsulo Ligamentous Repair in Chronic Scapho-Lunate Ligament Tears" by Prof. Christophe L. Mathoulin, MD, Nicolas Dauphin, MD, and Abhijeet L. Wahegaonkar, MBBS, D.Ortho, M.Ch (Ortho). We regret the error, and thank Dr Mathoulin and his co-authors for their manuscript submission, which will be included in the next issue, November 2011.

Hand Clinics

THE CLINICS ARE NOW AVAILABLE ONLINE!

Access your subscription at:
www.theclinics.com

Preface

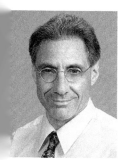

David J. Slutsky, MD
Guest Editor

Arthroscopy of the wrist and hand has evolved from being a mostly diagnostic modality to a valuable and effective therapeutic tool. There are so many new innovations that it was a struggle to limit the size of this issue to less than 20 articles, so the articles that are included consist of a choice pick of some of the best contributions from North America and overseas. Arthroscopy has revolutionized the diagnosis and treatment of wrist instability as well as the treatment of triangular fibrocartilage tears, which continues to evolve. Four separate articles on the diagnosis and treatment of foveal tears highlight the importance of this previously undertreated entity. Small joint arthroscopy of the CMC and MP joints has similarly undergone huge leaps in the diagnosis and treatment of small joint disorders. I greatly appreciate the time, effort, and personal sacrifice the contributors have put forth to educate their peers. I am also indebted to Deb Dellapena, who until recently has been at the helm of the *Hand Clinics* for over a decade. She has left a legacy which is to be admired. Special thanks to Katie Hartner, who has taken her place and brought this issue to completion.

This *Hand Clinics* is dedicated to my enduring best friends, my daughter Brett and my son Jesse. They continue to make me proud of who they have become.

David J. Slutsky, MD
The Hand and Wrist Institute
2808 Columbia Street
Torrance, CA 90503, USA

E-mail address:
d-slutsky@msn.com

Hand Clin 27 (2011) xiii
doi:10.1016/j.hcl.2011.06.006

All-Arthroscopic Repair of Peripheral Triangular Fibrocartilage Complex Tears Using FasT-Fix

Jeffrey Yao, MD

KEYWORDS

- Arthroscopy • Triangular fibrocartilage complex • TFCC
- FasT-Fix

The triangular fibrocartilage complex (TFCC) is an important dynamic stabilizer of the wrist. Studies have elucidated the importance of this structure with respect to rotation, translation, and load transmission at the wrist.[1–5] Injury to the TFCC is a major source of ulnar-sided wrist pain that results in disability with common activities of daily living involving forearm rotation.[6]

Palmer classified TFCC injuries into traumatic (type I) and degenerative (type II).[1] Specific to the scope of this article, a Palmer type IB lesion is defined as a traumatic injury to the ulnar attachment of the TFCC. This lesion involves a ligamentous avulsion from the ulnar capsule or fracture through the base of the ulnar styloid, resulting in distal radioulnar joint (DRUJ) instability and pain.[7]

With failure of conservative management, operative management is indicated. Repair of these tears is possible because of the excellent vascularity of the periphery of the TFCC. Past results with open repairs have been successful, but recent surgical advances have allowed a trend toward arthroscopic management. Arthroscopy allows improved visualization, decreased soft-tissue injury, decreased dissection of surrounding tissues, and improved final wrist motion.[8] Several arthroscopic methods have been described including inside-out, outside-in, and all-arthroscopic techniques.[9]

Recently, an all-arthroscopic technique of repair of Palmer type IB TFCC injuries with FasT-Fix suture technology (Smith and Nephew, Andover, MA, USA) has been described to be advantageous both biomechanically and in terms of decreasing risk of morbidity.[10]

CLINICAL PRESENTATION

The classic clinical presentation of a patient with a traumatic peripheral TFCC tear includes a history of a fall on to an outstretched, pronated wrist. Patients complain of ulnar-sided wrist pain, classically with activities involving forearm rotation, grip, and axial loads on the wrist. On physical examination, patients typically exhibit tenderness to direct palpation over the ulnar aspect of the wrist with positive TFCC grind and fovea signs. A palpable click is often present with a TFCC grind maneuver. Magnetic resonance imaging may be obtained for each individual to aid in the diagnosis of a TFCC injury. Nonoperative treatment regimens consist

This article was previously published in *Operative Techniques in Sports Medicine* 18:3.
Conflict of interest: The author has served as a consultant for Smith and Nephew Endoscopy in the past, but receives no royalties for the implant discussed in this article.
Department of Orthopaedic Surgery, Robert A. Chase Hand and Upper Limb Center, Stanford University Medical Center, 450 Broadway Street, Suite C-442, Redwood City, CA 94063, USA
E-mail address: jyao@stanford.edu

Hand Clin 27 (2011) 237–242
doi:10.1016/j.hcl.2011.05.004

of rest and immobilization, nonsteroidal anti-inflammatory drugs, physical therapy, and corticosteroid injections. If these modalities fail to improve the patient's ulnar-sided wrist symptoms, surgical treatment is indicated. Open, arthroscopic-assisted, and all-arthroscopic techniques have been described to adequately treat these injuries. The following novel technique is useful for those patients with refractory symptoms with or without concomitant DRUJ instability. Although this technique was initially used to repair peripheral TFCC tears without concomitant DRUJ instability, this capsular repair has also more recently been used to restore stability to the DRUJ, with success.

SURGICAL TECHNIQUE

A standard wrist arthroscopy tower is used with 10 to 12 lb of longitudinal traction placed on the index and long fingers to distract the radiocarpal joint. The standard 3–4 and 6R portals are used for diagnostic arthroscopy. After a peripheral (Palmer IB) tear is identified, it is debrided by use of a 3.5-mm full-radius motorized shaver to stimulate angiogenesis at the repair site (**Fig. 1**A–C). With the arthroscope in the 6R portal looking down at the periphery of the TFCC, the curved FasT-Fix (Smith & Nephew Endoscopy, Andover, MA, USA) is inserted through the 3–4 portal with the assistance of the split cannula and advanced into the ulnocarpal joint (see **Fig. 1**D). The first poly-L-lactic acid (PLLA) block is inserted radial to the tear and then advanced through the articular disc of the TFCC, and further advanced through the ulnar capsule. On penetration of the ulnar wrist capsule, a distinct decrease in resistance is felt. The needle introducer is then drawn back, releasing the block from the introducer and depositing the block on the outside of the ulnar wrist capsule. The trigger on the needle introducer is used to advance the second block into the deployment position. The second block is advanced and

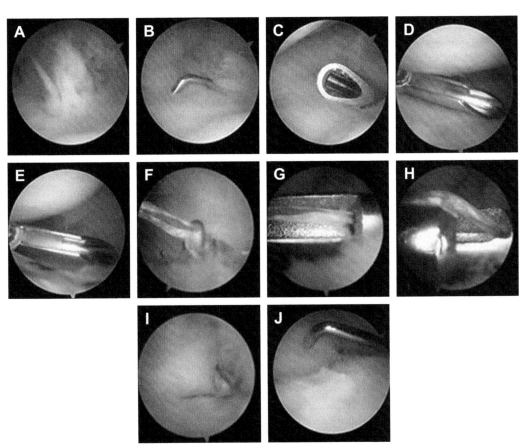

Fig. 1. All-arthroscopic TFCC repair with FasT-Fix. (*A*) Identification of Palmer type IB TFCC tear. (*B*) Demonstration of negative trampoline effect. (*C*) Debridement of TFCC tear to stimulate angiogenesis at repair site. (*D*) FasT-Fix inserted through 3–4 portal. (*E*) Second FasT-Fix block is advanced. (*F*) Needle introducer is removed from joint leaving pretied suture. (*G*) Suture is tightened with knot pusher/cutter. (*H*) Suture is cut by knot pusher/cutter. (*I*) Repair of Palmer type IB TFCC tear. (*J*) Evidence of positive trampoline test after repair.

deposited in the same fashion ulnar to the tear (approximately 3 mm from the first block), forming a vertical mattress configuration (see **Fig. 1**E). The needle introducer is removed from the joint, leaving the pretied suture (see **Fig. 1**F). The suture is tightened and the knot cut by use of the knot pusher/cutter (see **Fig. 1**G–I). Once the repair is completed, the strength of the repair may be evaluated using an arthroscopic probe. Adequate restoration of the trampoline effect should be achieved (see **Fig. 1**J). A second implant, if necessary, is placed adjacent (typically dorsal) to the initial implant. The stability of the DRUJ should also be confirmed. The wounds are closed with a monofilament suture, and the patient's extremity is placed into a well-molded sugar tong splint with the forearm in neutral rotation for 2 weeks. The first postoperative visit involves removal of the skin sutures and placement of a long arm Munster cast for an additional 4 weeks to allow elbow flexion and extension, but to prevent forearm rotation. Wrist range of motion exercises begin thereafter, with strengthening beginning at 8 weeks postoperatively.

INITIAL CLINICAL RESULTS

Recently, the author completed a retrospective review of patients treated using this technique from September 2005 to January 2009.[11] Fourteen patients who underwent FasT-Fix repairs were identified. Each individual sustained a traumatic injury, typically a fall on to an outstretched pronated wrist, and had a Palmer IB peripheral tear (diagnosed on arthroscopy) that failed nonoperative treatment. The patients' charts were reviewed for age, gender, injured side, hand dominance, location of tear, treatment, postoperative complications, range of motion, grip strength (percentage of contralateral), and return to full activity. In addition, each patient completed Quick Disabilities of the Arm, Shoulder, and Hand (*Quick* DASH) and Patient-Rated Wrist Evaluation (PRWE)

questionnaires. Statistical analysis was performed with linear regression correlations with significance set at $P<.05$.

The mean follow-up period was 16.1 months (range, 12–24 months). Mean supination was 81° ($\pm$13.1°, 15 patients, range 60°–90°) and the mean grip strength was 66% ($\pm$13.8%, 13 patients, range 38%–96%) of nonoperative extremity. All patients obtained supination and grip strength by 3 months after surgery (range 1–6 months). All other ranges of motion including pronation, flexion, extension, and radial and ulnar deviation were full at final follow-up for all patients.

The mean *Quick* DASH score was 10.2 ($\pm$11.4, 15 patients, range 0–43.2). The mean PRWE score was 18.8 ($\pm$13.5, 15 patients, range 2–52.5). The mean time to return to full activity and sports was 5.2 months (15 patients, range 2–9 months). There were no surgical complications of the procedure. No significant correlation was made between outcomes and age, gender, workers' compensation, disability status, or hand dominance. The only significant positive correlation was between the DASH and PRWE scores ($P = .0003$, $r = 0.82$, 95% confidence interval 0.52–0.94).

The one workers' compensation patient complained of persistent ulnar-sided wrist pain 12 months into the follow-up period and underwent an ulnar-shortening osteotomy (DASH 2.27, PRWE 11.5). Of note, arthroscopy at the time of the osteotomy revealed the TFCC tear had healed (**Fig. 2**). The trampoline effect was maintained. In addition, the suture had been completely encapsulated within 1 year. The patient's ulnar-sided wrist pain subsequently resolved after the ulnar-shortening osteotomy.

DISCUSSION

TFCC injuries are common, especially in an active patient population. When nonoperative modalities fail to resolve symptoms associated with this injury,

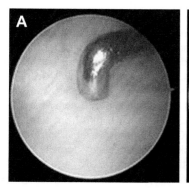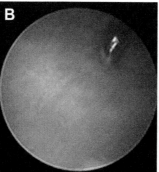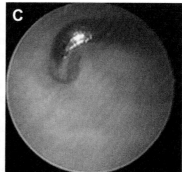

Fig. 2. Second look after all-arthroscopic TFCC repair. (*A*) Restoration of trampoline effect. (*B*) Suture has resorbed completely. (*C*) No evidence of tear with probing.

surgical management is indicated. Several open, arthroscopic-assisted, and arthroscopic techniques have been described.

Reiter and colleagues[12] reported on 46 patients treated with an inside-out arthroscopic repair. In this study, patients had a reduction in pain (mean preoperative visual analog score [VAS] of 7.5 vs postsurgical VAS of 3.4), and improvement in grip strength (mean 85% of contralateral extremity). Range of motion returned to 171 ± 19 pronation/supination arc. The average DASH score was 21.7 (±17.17) (range, 0–58.33).

Corso and colleagues[13] described results from a multicenter study using an arthroscopic-aided zone-specific repair. The technique incorporated an outside-in technique with 2-0 polydioxanone suture (PDS) with a small 1.5-cm incision over the head of the ulna. Results were graded according to the Mayo modified wrist score for total of 45 patients with 29 excellent, 12 good, 1 fair, and 3 poor. Range of motion returned to normal for all patients. Grip strength was at least 75% of the contralateral extremity.

Estrella and colleagues[14] described results from arthroscopic repair of a Palmer IB (11 patients), IC (5 patients), and ID (1 patient). This study used a zone-specific repair similar to the study by Corso and colleagues.[13] The modified Mayo wrist score was excellent in 54%, good in 20%, fair in 12%, and poor in 14%. Grip strength returned to 82% of the contralateral extremity and near full pronation/supination arc (98% pronation, 95% supination of contralateral extremity) was achieved.

The aforementioned studies are the largest-scale studies that critically examine results of arthroscopic treatment of TFCC tears. All 3 studies note the definitive value of arthroscopy with respect to diagnosis on direct visualization, minimization of soft-tissue trauma, cosmesis, and quicker recovery.[13–15]

Three other all-inside techniques have been described in recent literature.[15–17] The technique described by Conca and colleagues[17] uses a specialized small suture hook (Linvatec, Largo, FL, USA) that is inserted percutaneously perpendicular to the Palmer IB tear. The hook captures both sides of the lesion and allows a side-to-side repair of the lesion, similar to rotator cuff repairs. The investigators reported that all patients had an improvement in strength, pain, and range of motion. There was no mention of the number of patients or of complications associated with the procedure. The technique described by Pederzini and colleagues[15] involves making a 1.5-cm incision in the region of the 6U portal to avoid the sensory branch of the sensory nerve. A monofilament suture is passed through a slotted needle through the 6R portal

and an extra-articular loop is used to reapproximate the TFCC tear. The advantage to this technique is the placement of the knot within the joint, thereby avoiding residual ulnar pain from fixation of knot to the floor of the extensor carpi ulnaris (ECU) tendon sheath. In fact, this technique is essentially an outside-in technique with the knot placed inside the joint. By contrast, Bohringer and colleagues[16] described an all-inside technique similar to the author's, using similar tools from arthroscopic knee meniscal repairs. However, clinical results from using the double-T Mitek anchor (Mitek Worldwide, Westwood, MA, USA) and meniscal fastener have not yet been reported.

The current technique using the FasT-Fix provides additional benefits over other arthroscopic TFCC repairs by eliminating the need for separate incisions and challenging knot-tying. This technique also requires significantly less time to perform, and there are also no prominent suture knots that may act as subcutaneous irritants. Thus far, no patients have complained about the PLLA blocks that have been deposited on the outside of the ulnar capsule, likely because these implants have a low profile.

The author's recent retrospective study revealed excellent short-term and medium-term results. At minimum 1-year follow-up, 93% of the patients achieved excellent subjective outcomes based on *Quick* DASH and PRWE questionnaires, and on objective measurements of range of motion, similar to previous studies on TFCC repair. Also, the safety and biomechanical strength of the FasT-Fix repair have been studied in cadavers.[18] Compared with traditional outside-in techniques, the all-arthroscopic repair with FasT-Fix was stronger, with significantly greater load to failure (73.34 N) compared with outside-in 2-0 PDS monofilament sutures (55.77 N) (**Fig. 3**). The implants were also found to be a safe distance away from the at-risk neurovascular structures. The mean distance of the blocks from the ulnar neurovascular bundle was 1.8 cm, and 1.7 cm from the dorsal sensory branch of the ulnar nerve (DBUN). Waterman and colleagues[19] recently published a similar safety study regarding the use of this device, and found that the mean distance of the peripheral and central blocks were 4.2 mm and 9.6 mm away from the ECU tendon, respectively. The blocks were also found to be 3.8 mm and 6.8 mm away from the DBUN, and 8.3 mm and 7.6 mm from the flexor carpi ulnaris (FCU) tendon. However, in some specimens the blocks were placed very dorsally (placed very close to the ECU and DBUN), and therefore the investigators express concern regarding the safety of this technique when used routinely. The differences in the location of the implants found

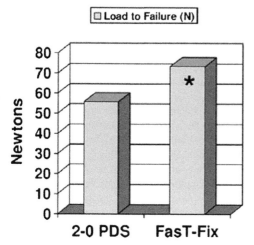

Fig. 3. Load to failure of FasT-Fix versus 2-0 PDS (*P<.05).

period and earlier return to competition but also an earlier, more accurate, and more complete diagnosis than other imaging techniques.

However, it must be noted that this recent change in the postoperative protocol was not specifically investigated in the author's retrospective study, so widespread use of this accelerated rehabilitation protocol cannot be recommended until the safety and positive outcomes of this protocol are confirmed through further study.

SUMMARY

This new technique of all-arthroscopic TFCC repair using the FasT-Fix has been shown to result in clinical outcomes that are comparable with previously described techniques. The potential benefits of this technique include its safety, ease of use, the decreased time necessary to complete a repair, and the elimination of extra incisions and irritating subcutaneous suture-knot stacks. Although the device carries a higher cost than other available techniques, the author believes this cost is mitigated by the shorter surgical time ($40 per minute at the author's institution) and the benefits of the decreased degree and duration of postoperative immobilization on the patients' quality of life. Perhaps the greatest benefit is associated with the greater biomechanical strength of the repair, which may allow decreased postoperative immobilization and accelerated rehabilitation protocols. Further study to elucidate this is ongoing and necessary.

ACKNOWLEDGMENTS

The author would like to thank Smith and Nephew for providing some of the materials used in developing this technique.

during these two studies highlight the potential variability of placement of these implants during this procedure. However, using the previously described technique, the author finds that the trajectory of the implant as it is introduced from the dorsal 3–4 portal must follow a dorsal to volar trajectory, which explains the more volar position of the blocks found in his study.[18] The author highly recommends following the natural dorsal to volar trajectory when using this implant to repair peripheral TFCC injuries. In his experience of using this implant clinically, the author has encountered no complications, with no instances of injury to the ECU, DBUN, ulnar neurovascular bundle, and FCU.

The recent strong data have encouraged the author to reduce postoperative immobilization and accelerate the rehabilitation protocol following these repairs.[18] The current protocol includes a short arm splint for the first 2 postoperative weeks followed by a short arm cast for an additional 2 weeks. Although forearm rotation is neither prohibited nor prevented with immobilization, patients are counseled to avoid forearm rotation during the first 4 weeks. Range of motion exercises of the wrist and forearm begin at 4 weeks postoperatively, with no restriction on forearm rotation. The elimination of elbow immobilization and reduced overall immobilization time has greatly improved the quality of life of the most recently treated patients. This schedule may be beneficial not just for the general population but also for the competitive athlete, for whom timing of return to play is crucial.[20] Whipple and Geissler[8] emphasized the true benefit of arthroscopic treatment of the TFCC as not only offering an abbreviated recuperation

REFERENCES

1. Palmer AK. Triangular fibrocartilage disorders: injury patterns and treatment. Arthroscopy 1990;6:125–32.
2. Palmer AK, Glisson RR, Werner FW. Relationship between ulnar variance and triangular fibrocartilage complex thickness. J Hand Surg Am 1984;9:681–2.
3. Palmer AK, Werner FW. The triangular fibrocartilage complex of the wrist—anatomy and function. J Hand Surg Am 1981;6:153–62.
4. Palmer AK, Werner FW. Biomechanics of the distal radioulnar joint. Clin Orthop Relat Res 1984;(187):26–35.
5. Palmer AK, Werner FW, Glisson RR, et al. Partial excision of the triangular fibrocartilage complex. J Hand Surg Am 1988;13:391–4.
6. Bain GI, Munt J, Turner PC. New advances in wrist arthroscopy. Arthroscopy 2008;24:355–67.

7. Henry MH. Management of acute triangular fibrocartilage complex injury of the wrist. J Am Acad Orthop Surg 2008;16:320–9.

8. Whipple TL, Geissler WB. Arthroscopic management of wrist triangular fibrocartilage complex injuries in the athlete. Orthopedics 1993;16:1061–7.

9. Chloros GD, Wiesler ER, Poehling GG. Current concepts in wrist arthroscopy. Arthroscopy 2008;24:343–54.

10. Yao J, Dantuluri P, Osterman AL. A novel technique of all-inside arthroscopic triangular fibrocartilage complex repair. Arthroscopy 2007;23:1357.e1–4.

11. Yao J, Lee AT. All-arthroscopic repair of Palmer 1B triangular fibrocartilage complex tears using the FasT-Fix device. J Hand Surg Am 2011;36(5):836–42.

12. Reiter A, Wolf MB, Schmid U, et al. Arthroscopic repair of Palmer 1B triangular fibrocartilage complex tears. Arthroscopy 2008;24:1244–50.

13. Corso SJ, Savoie FH, Geissler WB, et al. Arthroscopic repair of peripheral avulsions of the triangular fibrocartilage complex of the wrist: a multicenter study. Arthroscopy 1997;13:78–84.

14. Estrella EP, Hung LK, Ho PC, et al. Arthroscopic repair of triangular fibrocartilage complex tears. Arthroscopy 2007;23:729–37, 737.e1.

15. Pederzini LA, Tosi M, Prandini M, et al. All-inside suture technique for Palmer class 1B triangular fibrocartilage repair. Arthroscopy 2007;23:1130.e1–4.

16. Bohringer G, Schadel-Hopfner M, Petermann J, et al. A method for all-inside arthroscopic repair of Palmer 1B triangular fibrocartilage complex tears. Arthroscopy 2002;18:211–3.

17. Conca M, Conca R, Dalla Pria A. Preliminary experience of fully arthroscopic repair of triangular fibrocartilage complex lesions. Arthroscopy 2004;20:e79–82.

18. Yao J. All-arthroscopic triangular fibrocartilage complex repair: safety and biomechanical comparison with a traditional outside-in technique in cadavers. J Hand Surg Am 2009;34:671–6.

19. Waterman SM, Slade D, Masini BD, et al. Safety analysis of all-inside arthroscopic repair of peripheral triangular fibrocartilage complex. Arthroscopy 2010;26(11):1474–7.

20. McAdams TR, Swan J, Yao J. Arthroscopic treatment of triangular fibrocartilage wrist injuries in the athlete. Am J Sports Med 2009;37:291–7.

Radial Side (1D) Tears

Thomas Trumble, MD

KEYWORDS

- Triangular fibrocartilage complex (TFCC)
- Arthroscopic repairs • Wrist ligament
- Distal radioulnar joint (DRUJ) • Bone tunnels

PREOPERATIVE CONSIDERATIONS
Anatomy and Pathoanatomy

In 1989, Palmer and Werner coined the term triangular fibrocartilage complex (TFCC) to describe the set of related structures at the distal ulnar aspect of the wrist. The TFCC physically separates the distal radioulnar joint (DRUJ) from the radiocarpal joint. The TFCC must simultaneously be robust and flexible. It must have the strength to transmit 20% of the load of the carpus to the ulna and also to stabilize the DRUJ and ulnar carpus in conjunction with the bony architecture of the sigmoid notch. It must also be supple enough to accommodate the significant, complex motion that occurs during forearm rotation. The motion of the DRUJ is a combination of approximately 150° of rotation and sliding, which is caused by the 50% larger radius of curvature of the radial side of the DRUJ (15 mm vs 10 mm) (**Fig. 1**). The axis of rotation passes through the fovea of the ulnar head, which is a major attachment site for the TFCC. The 5 structures that comprise the TFCC are the articular disk; the distal radioulnar ligaments (both palmar and dorsal); the meniscal homolog; and the extensor carpi ulnaris subsheath, which is confluent with the (ulnocarpal collateral ligament).[1] The central portion of the complex consists of an articular disc called the triangular fibrocartilage (TFC). The disc is predominately composed of type II collagen, which is consistent with its role of distributing compressive forces. It lies in the axial plane and structurally represents an extension of the articular surface of the distal radius. Dorsally and palmarly, the TFC is surrounded by the radioulnar ligaments, which are transverse bands, which derive their broad origin from the sigmoid notch of the distal radius and insert on the base of the ulnar styloid.

The ulno-triquetral and ulno-lunate ligaments form the palmar border of the TFCC, and although Palmer and Werner did not include them in their original description of the TFCC, they serve an important role in the stability of the ulnar side of the wrist.

The ulnar and dorsal edges of the complex consist of the extensor carpi ulnaris (ECU) tendon subsheath and dorsal radial triquetral ligament, respectively. When viewed in the axial plane, these borders form a stout pyramid that attaches the TFCC to the ulnar side of the carpus. Stability of the TFCC is a prerequisite for smooth pronosupination and pain-free load bearing through the articular disc. The vestigial meniscal homolog derives from the synovium; its function is unclear, and it is often absent.

The blood supply of the TFCC enters from the periphery (**Fig. 2**). Thiru and colleagues[2] evaluated cadaveric specimens and found 3 main branches to the TFCC. The ulnar periphery of the TFCC has the richest blood supply and, consequently, the greatest potential for healing. It is fed predominantly via the dorsal and palmar radiocarpal branches of the ulnar artery. Dorsal and palmar branches of the anterior interosseous artery supply the more radial part of the complex.

CLASSIFICATION OF TFCC INJURIES

Palmer's original classification divides injuries of the TFCC into degenerative and acute tears (**Box 1**).[3] Furthermore, the classification is anatomically subdivided into radial, central, or ulnar tears. This classification bears consideration because the vascular anatomy dictates the healing potential and, therefore, the treatment and prognosis for TFCC tears, akin to the knee's meniscus.

Bellevue Bone and Joint Physicians, Affiliate Physician Overlake Hospital Medical Center, Department of Orthopaedic Surgery, 1632 116th Avenue NE #C, Bellevue, WA 98040, USA
E-mail address: t.trumble@comcast.net

Hand Clin 27 (2011) 243–254
doi:10.1016/j.hcl.2011.05.013
0749-0712/11/$ – see front matter © 2011 Published by Elsevier Inc.

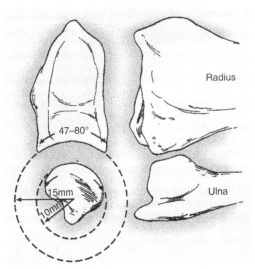

Fig. 1. The radius of curvature of the sigmoid notch is 1.5 to 2.0 times that of the ulnar head. (*From* Adams BD. The distal radioulnar joint and triangular fibrocartilage complex. In: Trumble TE, editor. Principles of hand surgery and therapy. 2nd edition. Philadelphia: Elsevier; 2010. p. 119; Fig. 6–1; with permission.)

Class 1: These acute, traumatic injuries are subdivided into 4 types based on the site of injury (see **Box 1**).

> *Type 1A* lesions involve the central avascular portion; the rim is still attached to the radius. This lesion is generally not amenable to direct repair. Arthroscopic treatment is limited to debridement of the central tear to remove any flaps that may impede movement.
>
> *Type 1B* (ulnar-avulsion) lesions are peripheral tears that occur when the ulnar side of the

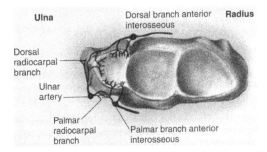

Fig. 2. Only the periphery of the triangular fibrocartilage disc receives blood directly. Vascular perforators from the radius supply the radial margin of the TFCC. (*From* Adams BD. The distal radioulnar joint and triangular fibrocartilage complex. In: Trumble TE, editor. Principles of hand surgery and therapy. 2nd edition. Philadelphia: Elsevier; 2010. p. 119, Fig. 6–1; with permission.)

Box 1
Classification of TFCC injury

Class 1: Traumatic
1. Central perforation
2. Ulnar avulsion
   a. With distal ulnar fracture
   b. Without distal ulnar fracture
3. Distal avulsion
4. Radial avulsion
   a. With sigmoid notch fracture
   b. Without sigmoid notch fracture

Class 2: Degenerative (ulnocarpal abutment syndrome)
1. Stage
   a. TFCC wear
   b. TFCC wear
      i. Lunate or ulnar chondromalacia
   c. TFCC perforation
      i. Lunate or ulnar chondromalacia
   d. TFCC perforation
      i. Lunate or ulnar chondromalacia
      ii. Lunotriquetral ligament perforation
   e. TFCC perforation
      i. Lunate or ulnar chondromalacia
      ii. Lunotriquetral ligament perforation
      iii. Ulnocarpal arthritis

Data from Palmer AK. Triangular fibrocartilage complex lesions: a classification. J Hand Surg Am 1989;14:594–606.

TFCC complex is avulsed from its capsule and can be associated with ulnar styloid fractures.

> *Type 1C* (ulnar-distal) injuries involve ruptures along the volar attachment of the TFCC or distal ulnocarpal ligaments; this is variably amenable to repair.
>
> *Type 1D* (radial-avulsion) injuries are rare injuries with tears from the radial attachment. These injuries represent traumatic avulsions of the TFCC from the attachment at the sigmoid notch, with or without a fracture of the sigmoid notch. **Fig. 3** Type 1D injuries often occur in young, active athletes with traumatic injuries.

Class 2: Degenerative TFCC lesions all involve the central portion and are staged from *A* to *E*, depending on the presence or absence of a TFCC

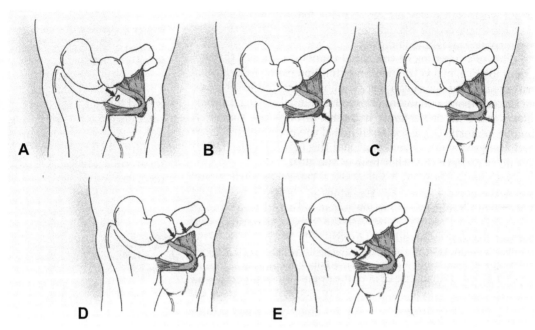

Fig. 3. Repairable lesions of the triangular fibrocartilage complex include Palmer class 1B, 1C, and 1D. (*A*) Class 1A radial-sided perforation (not repairable). (*B*) Class B ulnar-sided lesion with avulsion of the TFCC from the ulnar styloid or (*C*) class 1B lesion with destabilization of the TFCC caused by fractures of the ulnar styloid. (*D*) Class 1C lesion with avulsion of the ulnolunate and ulnotriquetral ligaments. (*E*) Class 1D lesion with avulsion of the radial attachment of the TFCC, including the dorsal and palmar origins of the radioulnar ligaments. The arrows note the location of the tear of the triangular fibrocartilage. (*From* Adams BD. The distal radioulnar joint and triangular fibrocartilage complex. In: Trumble TE, editor. Principles of hand surgery and therapy. 2nd edition. Philadelphia: Elsevier; 2010. p. 126, Fig. 6–19; with permission.)

perforation, lunate and ulnar chondromalacia, lunotriquetral ligament perforation, or degenerative radiocarpal arthritis. These degenerative lesions usually arise from ulnar abutment. Generally, class 2 lesions are not amenable to surgical repair and are treated with debridement.

TFCC tears can be further subdivided by their acuity. Acute tears are from 0 to 3 months, subacute tears are 3 months to 1 year, and chronic tears present with typically greater than 1 year of symptoms. The chronicity has prognostic implications; generally, addressing tears in the acute phase provides better results.[4–6]

MECHANISM OF INJURY, HISTORY, SIGNS, AND SYMPTOMS

Ulnar-sided wrist pain has been referred to as the low back pain of the hand surgeon. The multitude of structures and diagnoses that can contribute to patients' symptoms are often subtle and require precise physical examination and correlation with history and imaging.

A typical history for an acute TFCC tear involves a fall on an outstretched hand or forced forearm rotation. The literature is controversial over which ligaments are tightest in varying positions of forearm supination or pronation, but nevertheless, an acute or delayed complaint of ulnar-sided wrist pain, often radiating dorsally, exacerbated by firm grasp and push off (wrist extended, getting up from a table) are characteristic features of a patient's history. One report suggests that injuries can occur in either pronation or supination and the mechanism results in different patterns of ligament injuries.[7] Achiness with repetitive supination and pronation tasks is also common. The pain is often characterized as diffuse, deep, and sometimes burning.

Chronic attritional injuries and degenerative changes of the ulnocarpal joint, including the TFCC, result from repetitive overloading. Ulnar deviation of the wrist, along with forearm supination and power grasp, increase the damage from axial loads. Patients with acquired ulnar positive variance, discussed in greater detail later, are at a higher risk for degenerative changes and recurrent injury from minor trauma.

A clicking sensation may be present with wrist pronation and supination. Patients may also complain of generalized weakness both with and without wrist loading. Importantly, patients often delay treatment or are misdiagnosed as having a wrist sprain that fails to improve.

TFCC tears have also been associated with distal radius fractures on imaging and direct arthroscopy. The incidence varies in different studies, but ranges between 13% and 60%.[8–11] Unfortunately, the literature is not clear in the absence of frank DRUJ instability, which tears should be fixed and by which methods. This lack of clarity is partly because it is unclear how many of these tears become symptomatic. Likely, many of these tears are effectively treated by the treatment of the concomitant fracture.[8] Nevertheless, several investigators have endorsed the technique of using arthroscopy to fix distal radius fractures and to identify and treat concomitant soft-tissue injuries. A recent report by Varitimidis and colleagues[11] found that 60% of their patients with distal radius fracture had TFCC tears, half of which were ulnar sided. All TFCC tears underwent debridement; 20% (2 of 12) had arthroscopic repair and 1 patient required open repair. The arthroscopic group demonstrated improved range of motion and Mayo wrist scores versus the nonarthroscopic group, treated with traditional external fixation. Ruch and colleagues[12] demonstrated good to excellent results with the acute repair of the TFCC at the time of distal radius operative treatment in 56 patients, with only 2 patients with transient ulnar dorsal sensory irritation, but the study lacked a control group.

Lindau and colleagues[13] reported that 10 of 11 patients with a documented complete peripheral TFCC tear associated with a distal radius fracture exhibited DRUJ instability at a 1-year follow-up examination versus 22% with no peripheral tears or only partial tears. This instability was correlated with worse clinical outcomes.

Physical Examination

Acute TFCC injuries frequently present with ulnar-sided wrist swelling that may reverse the normal convex shape of the ulnar wrist border. The soft, ballotable region between the ulnar styloid and the triquetrum can frequently be point tender. (**Fig. 4**) Clicking can often be elicited with passive and active circumduction of the wrist. The specialized tests to distinguish TFCC injuries from other ulnar wrist injuries include the TFCC compression test, ulnar impaction test, and the piano key test. Significant pain from axial loading of the TFCC in conjunction with ulnar deviation is a positive compression test. Similarly, pain with the combination of wrist hyperextension and the previous maneuvers is a positive ulnar impaction test.[14]

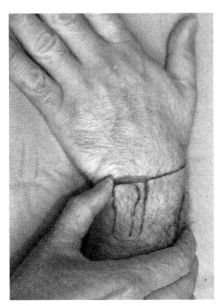

Fig. 4. Physical examination with tenderness along the ulnar border of the wrist especially with ulnar deviation is key maneuver to diagnose TFCC injuries.

Comparing any dorsal-volar plane instability of the DRUJ to the normal contralateral side is the piano key test. This test should be performed in neutral, supination, and pronation. The DRUJ typically has the most anterior-posterior translation in the neutral position. Furthermore, volar subluxation of the distal ulna with wrist supination can be appreciated by dimpling of the skin of the dorsal ulnar border (**Fig. 5**). A lunotriquetral ballottement test is performed to test lunotriquetral ligament stability, and pisotriquetral manipulation should be performed to rule out arthrosis of this joint.

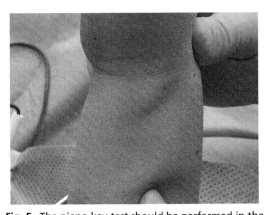

Fig. 5. The piano key test should be performed in the neutral, supination, and pronation position. The DRUJ typically has the most anterior-posterior translation in the neutral position. Volar subluxation of the distal ulna with wrist supination can be appreciated by dimpling of the skin of the dorsal ulnar border.

Diagnostic Imaging

Ulnar-sided wrist pain of acute or chronic nature warrants posteroanterior (PA), lateral, and oblique radiographs of the wrist. With true neutral rotation, PA radiographs are taken with the shoulder in 90° of abduction and the elbow in 90° of flexion. The ulnar styloid should be visible at the far ulnar portion of the distal ulna in a true posteroanterior view, whereas it is seen in the mid portion of the distal ulna with radiographs taken in a supinated or pronated position. The pisiform should lie between the palmar surface of the scaphoid distal pole and the capitate in a true lateral view.

Ulnar variance is the difference between the length of the ulna and the length of the radius at the ulnar side of the radiocarpal joint. Specifically, this distance is measured between lines drawn perpendicular to the shaft of the radius and the ulna corner of the radius and a line drawn along the distal articular surface of the ulna. An ulnar positive or negative variance is defined as the distal ulna being longer or shorter, respectively, than the radius. This point is clinically important for several reasons. Anatomically, Palmer[15] has shown that the ulnar variance is inversely correlated with the thickness of the central portion of the TFC. In addition, cystic changes in the lunate and distal ulna, especially in conjunction with an ulnar neutral or positive variance, can be the hallmark of excessive loading through the ulnar carpus, as is the case with ulnar impaction syndrome. These changes may suggest the need for off-loading procedures, such as an ulnar shortening osteotomy in conjunction with TFCC treatment. In this setting, investigators have shown encouraging results combining these treatments. Trumble and colleagues[6] demonstrated significant relief of pain. Grip strength and range of motion both averaged approximately 80% of the uninjured side. Furthermore, central TFCC tears treated in the setting of the ulnar positive variance with ulnar shortening osteotomy alone have shown 50% healing on second-look arthroscopy, with a spectrum of greatest-to-least healing on the more vascular ulnar side as compared with the less vascular radial side.[16]

Plain films

Plain radiographs are undoubtedly important to rule out alternative causes of wrist pain, but the correlation between specific radiographic findings and injuries to the TFCC itself remains contentious. Geissler and colleagues[8–10,17] concluded that TFCC tear occurred in the 26 of 60 patients in their series which was the most common intracarpal soft tissue lesion that they found. He thought radiographs were most helpful in scapholunate ligament injuries but the least helpful in TFCC tears. Despite this finding, radiographic findings of a DRUJ dislocation or ulnar styloid fracture were the best surrogates to infer TFCC injury. Of the 25 patients with ulnar styloid fracture, 16 had TFCC tears, 14 of which were ulnar sided.[9,10] This finding was corroborated by Lindau and colleagues.[18] On the other hand, Richards and colleagues[19] found no correlation between ulnar styloid fractures and TFCC injuries. Instead, tears were related to greater shortening and dorsal angulation of the distal radius on the preoperative radiographs in his study of 118 intraarticular and extra-articular wrist fractures. In a 2008 study by Bombaci comparing magnetic resonance imaging (MRI) findings of TFCC tears with plain radiographs,[20] MRI revealed that 27 of the 60 patients (45%) had triangular fibrocartilage lesions. No correlation was found between a TFCC injury and the Melone classification system, the presence of an ulnar styloid fracture, comminution of the articular surface of the distal radius, greater than 20° of dorsal angulation of the distal radius, or subluxation/dislocation of the distal radioulnar joint on the plain radiographs. However, subtypes of distal radius fractures that extended into either the DRUJ or the radiocarpal joint and included an ulnar styloid fracture did have a statistically higher incidence of triangular fibrocartilage complex tears compared with the remaining Frykman subtypes injuries after distal radial fractures.

Arthrograms

Wrist arthrography can be used to help diagnose tears of the scapholunate and lunotriquetral interosseous ligaments.[21–24] Following a midcarpal row injection, the contrast is injected into the radiocarpal joint. Contrast extravasation into the distal radioulnar joint is indicative of the perforation of the TFCC (**Fig. 6**). Injecting directly into the DRUJ can demonstrate smaller tears or those with an overlying flap. Arthrograms more reliably diagnose TFCC radial detachment and lunotriquetral ligament tears than ulnocarpal ligament injuries and ulnar TFCC detachments.[7–9] In addition, single injection arthrograms have been shown to have a high incidence of positive findings in asymptomatic patients.[21] As always, it is important to correlate the presences of symptoms with the suspected findings on the study.

MRI

MRI for the diagnosis of TFCC injuries is a controversial issue. The specificity and sensitivity of MRI for detecting central and radial detachment vary, but can be improved by dedicated musculoskeletal

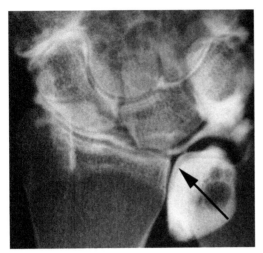

Fig. 6. The dye leakage (*arrow*) from the radial carpal joint into the distal radioulnar joint on an arthrogram helps to confirm a TFCC tear.

radiologists and specialized equipment, such as wrist surface coils and higher tesla magnets[25] (**Fig. 7**). Golimbu, Joshy, and Skahen[26–28] detected TFCC injuries with an accuracy between 74% and 95%.[26–28] Specifically in Joshy's study in which patients underwent arthroscopy following MRI arthrography, the positive predictive value was 0.95. They recommended viewing negative results with caution because the negative predictive value was only 0.50. This study unfortunately used a 1.0 T magnet, whereas a recent Mayo clinic study using 3.0 T magnets showed improved accuracy.[29] Furthermore, MRI appears to under stage some TFCC pathology, specifically the palmar radioulnar ligament and dorsal radioulnar ligament, while over staging others (radial-sided and disc tears) compared with arthroscopy for definitive diagnosis.[25,30] In the author's experience, the use of MR arthrograms have been the most efficient

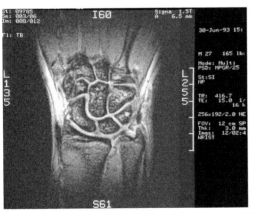

Fig. 7. The MRI demonstrates a signal change on a T-2 weighted images at the TFCC peripheral attachment.

and accurate nonoperative method of evaluating ulnar wrist pain.

INDICATIONS FOR SURGERY

The appropriate treatment for TFCC injuries varies and depends on the type of injury as well as the stability of the DRUJ and ulnar-sided carpus. If the patient history and physical examination are consistent with a TFCC injury, but the patients' have normal radiographs and clinical stability, and only mild symptoms, immobilization in a long-arm cast or brace for 3 to 4 weeks is usually successful. Other nonoperative measures include corticosteroid injections and nonsteroidal antiinflammatory medications. The author prefers to avoid steroid injection in young, active athletes. If patients continue to have pain after 1 month of conservative treatment, further diagnostic studies, such as arthrogram, MRI, or arthroscopy are warranted. Currently, the author recommends the use of an MR arthrogram as the most sensitive and accurate diagnostic study. Early evaluation is warranted in young, active patients with a history of significant injury and swelling on physical examination. If patients present with radiographic or clinical instability, arthroscopic evaluation and repair should be considered primarily.

Treatment

Indications for arthroscopic surgery
Patients with TFCC tears that fail to respond to nonoperative therapy for greater than 1 month, or in the presence of DRUJ instability, warrant operative intervention. TFCC lesions can be divided into radial or ulnar detachments, with their specific approaches detailed later, or central attritional tears that are amenable to debridement.

1. Repairable tears of the TFCC: Peripheral tears, such as type 1B, 1C, and 1D, do exceptionally well, partly because of their excellent blood supply. Techniques for repairing type 1B tears along the ulnar border have been demonstrated by numerous investigators. Arthroscopic repair techniques of type 1D tears are continuing to be honed.
2. Nonrepairable tears of the TFCC: Central degenerative tears and central tears that have a small rim attached to the radius (type 1A) usually cannot be repaired. In certain cases, the body of the TFCC can be advanced to the sigmoid notch and repaired similar to a type 1D lesion. In these cases, the torn rim along the sigmoid notch can be excised and the major body of the TFCC can be advanced and sutured to the radius.

3. Preferred open treatment: Specifically, TFCC injuries that are less amenable to arthroscopic intervention, in which an open approach should be considered, are those with combined ECU tendon instability, a large ulnar styloid avulsion fracture that requires open reduction and internal fixation to reestablish the primary ulnar attachment of the TFCC, and those patients with concomitant lunotriquetral or other intercarpal instability.

SURGICAL TECHNIQUES FOR ARTHROSCOPIC REPAIR OF 1D TFCC TEARS
Equipment and Implants

Required
Standard traction apparatus, such as wrist distraction tower

Small joint arthroscope 2.7 mm (1.9 mm for small female patients) with pressure monitoring system

Arthroscopic shaver, preferred 2.5 mm diameter with full radius blade

Small probe

Small arthroscope grasping and basket forceps

Wire suture grasper

Small hypodermic needle

18-gauge needle

Suction tip cannula

Small retractor

0.045-in Kirschner wire

2–0 Maxon meniscal repair sutures

3–0 Dacron sutures

Bioabsorbable suture anchor (Panalok Loop, Ethicon Inc, Norwood, MA, USA)

Small-joint radio-frequency device for capsular shrinkage or ablation

2.5-mm drill guide

Mini arthroscopic lasso (Arthrex, Naples, FL, USA)

Mini Pushlock (Arthrex, Naples, FL, USA) and 2–0 Fiberstick suture (Arthrex, Naples, FL, USA)

Positioning

The repairs are performed with patients supine using a wrist traction tower that positions the wrist and forearm vertically on the hand table. The arm is positioned so that a C-arm can be used for fluoroscopy during the procedure, if needed.

Procedure

This technique was modified from the technique described by Cooney[31] for open repairs using sutures placed through the radius. A wrist distraction tower is used to support the wrist, and the portals are marked out. (**Figs. 8** and **9**). A probe placed in the 4,5 portal is used to identify the tear (**Fig. 10**). The 2.5-mm full-radius, small-joint debrider is used with the mini-arthroscopic shaver

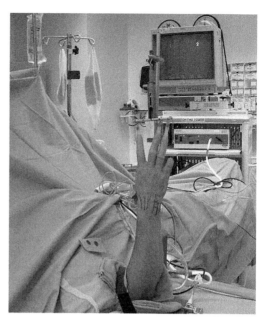

Fig. 8. The arm is positioned in a wrist arthroscopy tower with 10 to 15 lb of longitudinal traction.

for preparation of the reattachment of the TFCC. The mini-arthroscopic shaver can be placed through the 4,5 or the 6-U portal. The reattachment site of the TFCC on the distal radius is debrided down to the bleeding bone using an arthroscopic shaver or burr (**Fig. 11**).

After the tear has been identified and debrided, an 18-gage hypodermic needle is placed into the wrist joint through the 6-U portal. The needle tip will determine the appropriate access point for introducing the repair sutures (**Fig. 12**). The 6-U portal is located on the ulnar aspect of the ECU just proximal to the triquetrum. A small incision is then made in the region of the 6-U portal and blunt

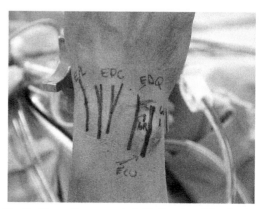

Fig. 9. The arthroscope is initially placed in the 3,4 portal and the probe is placed in the 4,5 portal to evaluate for TFCC tears.

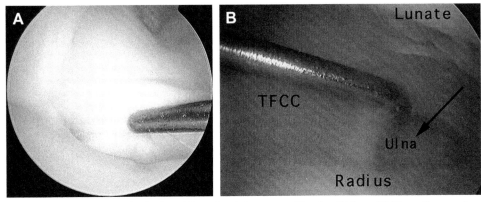

Fig. 10. (*A*) The arthroscopic probe is placed into the defect caused by the 1D tear. (*B*) The arthroscopic probe is elevating a large 1D tear. The arrow point to the head of the exposed ulna.

dissection is carried down to the bone to avoid injuries to the dorsal sensory branch of the ulnar nerve (**Fig. 13**). A cannula is inserted into the 6-U portal. This cannula can either be a drill guide or a second 2.7-mm arthroscopy cannula. Meniscal repair sutures (2–0 Maxon, Davis & Geck, Manati, Pennsylvania) are passed into the suction tip cannula, placed into the radial rim of the TFCC under arthroscopic guidance, and driven across the radius using a power wire driver (**Fig. 14**). Care is taken to avoid suture coiling when using this double-armed meniscal repair suture. When the first needle is passed, coiling is prevented by holding the suture and allowing the second needle to rotate. The second needle has to be inserted into the wire driver with the attached suture folded alongside the suture needle. A curved retractor is placed around the loop of the suture between

the tip of the wire driver and the patient. The suture coils along the needle as the needle is driven across the radius. Once the suture has coiled along the length of the needle, the direction of the wire driver is reversed. This procedure is continued until the needle exits the skin along the radial side of the wrist (**Fig. 15**). The suture needles should exit between the first and second dorsal compartments on the radial aspect of the wrist. The first suture is brought out through the skin and then the second suture is passed through the radius. Generally, 2 sets of repair sutures are used to secure the TFCC to the radius. The sutures are then placed under tension to ensure that the TFCC lines up with the surface of the distal radius. Once correct positioning of the TFCC has been confirmed, the patient's hand is removed from the traction device and an incision is made

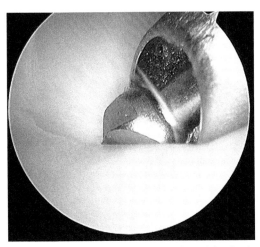

Fig. 11. An arthroscopic burr is used to debride the margin of the sigmoid notch down to bleeding bone, which is important to provide a vascular bed for the TFCC repair.

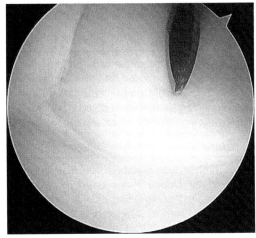

Fig. 12. The 18-gage needle is used to mark the correct orientation for the 6-U portal (ulnar to the ECU).

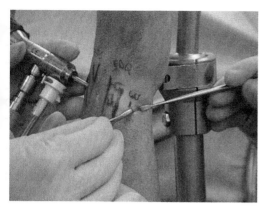

Fig. 13. The 6-U portal is located on the ulnar aspect of the ECU just proximal to the triquetrum. A small incision is then made in the region of the 6-U portal, and blunt dissection is carried down to bone to avoid the injuries to the dorsal sensory branch of the ulnar nerve.

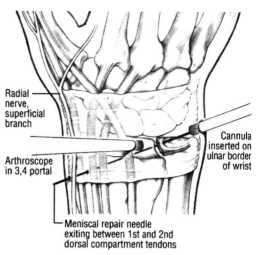

Fig. 15. The meniscal repair needles are drilled through the radius and brought out the radial border of the distal radius between the first and second compartments.

longitudinally between the 2 sets of exiting sutures. The extensor tendons in the first and second compartments are identified and retracted so that the suture can be placed under tension and tied onto the radius with the wrist in neutral rotation.

An alternative to the technique of drilling 2 holes, which can be difficult in a small wrist, is to use a cannulated 2.0-mm drill (Synthes Inc, Paoli, PA, USA) to drill a single hole from the sigmoid notch to the base of the radial styloid. The guide pin is drilled first through the 6-U portal with the 2.0-mm guide inserted into the wrist joint. The radial-sided incision is made once the exit site of the guide pin has been determined. The double-

armed sutures are passed through the cannula and through the TFCC. The sutures are secured by placing an absorbable anchor (Panalok Loop, Ethicon Inc, Norwood, MA, USA) between the sutures for an interference fit (**Fig. 16**). The sutures are then tied over the anchor (**Fig. 17**). In addition, new techniques are being developed that use a mini Pushlock anchor employing a fully arthroscopic technique. This technique can be facilitated by using the mini suture lasso and small arthroscopic cannulas to assist in passing the anchor into the sigmoid notch (**Fig. 18**). The key is to use a cannula or drill guide that is large enough to allow the mini Pushlock to be deployed through the 6-U portal. The 2–0 Fiberstick sutures are used in place of the more fragile bioabsorbable suture.

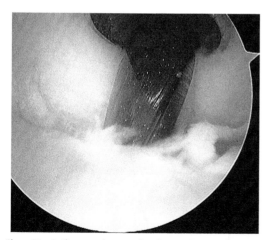

Fig. 14. Arthroscopic meniscal repair needles are placed through the 6-U portal and placed through the radial rim of the TFCC and drilled across the radius.

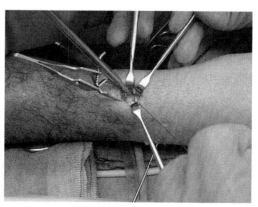

Fig. 16. A bioabsorbable anchor is used to provide an interference fit when a single drill hole is used to pass the TFCC repair sutures.

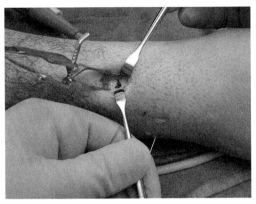

Fig. 17. The repair sutures are tied over the interference-fit anchor to secure the repair.

Results

Estrella's 2007 study only had 1 of 35 patients with a type 1D tear. Results were not given for that patient specifically.[32] In Shih's 2002 study, 8 of the patients had repairs of type 1D tears and "showed the same results" as those with type IB tears in this study of 37 patients with a 2-year follow-up with Mayo wrist scores.[33] The arthroscopic repair of acute injuries results in the recovery of 80% of the grip strength and range of motion compared with the contralateral side. (**Fig. 19**).[6] Trumble and colleagues[6] showed that,

postoperatively, there was a significant relief of pain. Postoperative range of motion averaged 89% (9% standard deviation [SD]) of the contralateral side, and grip strength averaged 85% (20% SD) of the contralateral side.

Osterman presented his results on a retrospective study of 19 patients with Palmer class 1D TFCC lesions without DRUJ instability that compared the clinical outcomes after TFCC reattachment versus debridement.[34] They concluded that debridement was equally effective as repair in alleviating wrist pain, improving grip strength, and restoring range of motion.

REHABILITATION

After a TFCC repair is performed, an above-elbow splint applied with the wrist in a neutral position should restrict the forearm rotation and wrist motion. Maintain the splint for 3 to 4 weeks and begin finger range-of-motion exercises during this period. After the long arm splint is removed, a removable wrist brace is used for an additional 2 weeks (postoperative weeks 4–6). Active wrist and forearm motion can be started at this time, but radial and ulnar deviation should be avoided to protect the repair. Generally, flexion and extension are permitted at 4 weeks, and supination and pronation are permitted slightly later at 6 weeks. Passive wrist range-of-motion exercises are

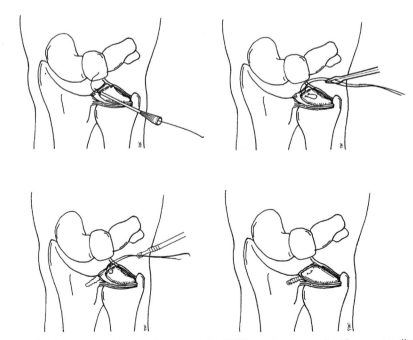

Fig. 18. A mini-Pushlock anchor can be used to secure the TFCC repair sutures. An 18-gage needle is used to pass the sutures that are retrieved with a mini-arthroscopic suture lasso. A mini Pushlock is inserted into a predrilled hole.

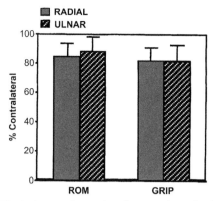

Fig. 19. Arthroscopic repairs of acute triangular fibrocartilage complex tears have resulted in the return of 80% of the grip strength and range of motion (ROM) of the contralateral uninjured wrist. (*From* Trumble TE, Gilbert M, Vedder N. Isolated tears of the triangular fibrocartilage: management by early arthroscopic repair. J Hand Surg Am 1997;22:57–65; with permission.)

started (postoperative weeks 6–8) followed by strengthening (postoperative weeks 8–12). Overall, the period of immobilization is adjusted for severity of injury, strength of repair, and patient compliance.

SUMMARY

For patients with wrist injuries that do not respond to an initial conservative treatment with splinting, MR arteriogram can provide an accurate diagnosis, especially in the setting of acute trauma in active patients. Type 1D lesions cause a major disruption in the articular contact between the distal ulna and the carpus. Arthroscopic repair of type ID lesions can allow for significant recovery of strength and motion to help the patients return to their work and sports activities.

REFERENCES

1. DiTano O, Trumble TE, Tencer AF. Biomechanical function of the distal radioulnar and ulnocarpal wrist ligaments. J Hand Surg 2003;28(4):622–7.
2. Thiru RG, Ferlic DC, Clayton ML, et al. Arterial anatomy of the triangular fibrocartilage of the wrist and its surgical significance. J Hand Surg Am 1986;11(2):258–63.
3. Palmer A. Triangular fibrocartilage complex lesions: a classification. J Hand Surg Am 1989;14(4):594–606.
4. Trumble T, Gilbert M, Vedder N. Arthroscopic repair of the triangular fibrocartilage complex. Arthroscopy 1996;12(5):588–97.
5. Trumble T, Gilbert M, Vedder N. Ulnar shortening combined with arthroscopic repairs in the delayed management of triangular fibrocartilage complex tears. J Hand Surg Am 1997;22(5):807–13.
6. Trumble T, Gilbert M, Vedder N. Isolated tears of the triangular fibrocartilage: management by early arthroscopic repair. J Hand Surg Am 1997;22(1):57–65.
7. Moritomo H, Masatomi T, Murase T, et al. Open repair of foveal avulsion of the triangular fibrocartilage complex and comparison by types of injury mechanism. J Hand Surg Am 2010;35(12):1955–63.
8. Geissler WB. Intra-articular distal radius fractures: the role of arthroscopy? Hand Clin 2005;21(3):407–16.
9. Geissler WB, Fernandez DL, Lamey DM. Distal radioulnar joint injuries associated with fractures of the distal radius. Clin Orthop Relat Res 1996;(327):135–46.
10. Geissler WB, Freeland AE, Savoie FH, et al. Intracarpal soft-tissue lesions associated with an intra-articular fracture of the distal end of the radius. J Bone Joint Surg Am 1996;78(3):357–65.
11. Varitimidis SE, Basdekis GK, Dailiana ZH, et al. Treatment of intra-articular fractures of the distal radius: fluoroscopic or arthroscopic reduction? J Bone Joint Surg Br 2008;90(6):778–85.
12. Ruch DS, Yang CC, Smith BP. Results of acute arthroscopically repaired triangular fibrocartilage complex injuries associated with intra-articular distal radius fractures. Arthroscopy 2003;19(5):511–6.
13. Lindau T, Adlercreutz C, Aspenberg P. Peripheral tears of the triangular fibrocartilage complex cause distal radioulnar joint instability after distal radial fractures. J Hand Surg Am 2000;25(3):464–8.
14. deAraujo W, Poehling G, Kuzma G. New Tuohy needle technique for triangular fibrocartilage complex repair: preliminary studies. Arthroscopy 1996;12(6):699–703.
15. Palmer AK, Glisson RR, Werner FW. Relationship between ulnar variance and triangular fibrocartilage complex thickness. J Hand Surg Am 1984;9(5):681–2.
16. Tatebe M, Horii E, Nakao E, et al. Repair of the triangular fibrocartilage complex after ulnar-shortening osteotomy: second-look arthroscopy. J Hand Surg Am 2007;32(4):445–9.
17. Geissler WB. Arthroscopically assisted reduction of intra-articular fractures of the distal radius. Hand Clin 1995;11(1):19–29.
18. Lindau T, Arner M, Hagberg L. Intraarticular lesions in distal fractures of the radius in young adults. A descriptive arthroscopic study in 50 patients. J Hand Surg Br 1997;22(5):638–43.
19. Richards RS, Bennett JD, Roth JH, et al. Arthroscopic diagnosis of intra-articular soft tissue injuries associated with distal radial fractures. J Hand Surg Am 1997;22(5):772–6.
20. Bombaci H, Polat A, Deniz G, et al. The value of plain X-rays in predicting TFCC injury after distal radial fractures. J Hand Surg Eur Vol 2008;33(3):322–6.
21. Brown J, Janzen D, Adler B, et al. Arthrography of the contralateral, asymptomatic wrist in patients

with unilateral wrist pain. Can Assoc Radiol J 1994; 45(4):292–6.

22. Cerofolini E, Luchetti R, Pederzini L, et al. MR evaluation of triangular fibrocartilage complex tears in the wrist: comparison with arthrography and arthroscopy. J Comput Assist Tomogr 1990;14(6):963–7.

23. Levinsohn EM, Palmer AK, Coren AB, et al. Wrist arthrography: the value of the three compartment injection technique. Skeletal Radiol 1987;16(7):539–44.

24. Levinsohn E, Rosen I, Palmer A. Wrist arthrography: value of the three-compartment injection method. Radiology 1991;179(1):231–9.

25. Tanaka T, Yoshioka H, Ueno T, et al. Comparison between high-resolution MRI with a microscopy coil and arthroscopy in triangular fibrocartilage complex injury. J Hand Surg Am 2006;31(8):1308–14.

26. Golimbu C, Firooznia H, Melone CJ, et al. Tears of the triangular fibrocartilage of the wrist: MR imaging. Radiology 1989;173(3):731–3.

27. Joshy S, Ghosh S, Lee K, et al. Accuracy of direct magnetic resonance arthrography in the diagnosis of triangular fibrocartilage complex tears of the wrist. Int Orthop 2008;32(2):251–3.

28. Skahen JI, Palmer A, Levinsohn E, et al. Magnetic resonance imaging of the triangular fibrocartilage complex. J Hand Surg Am 1990;15(4):552–7.

29. Anderson ML, Skinner JA, Felmlee JP, et al. Diagnostic comparison of 1.5 tesla and 3.0 tesla preoperative MRI of the wrist in patients with ulnar-sided wrist pain. J Hand Surg Am 2008;33(7):1153–9.

30. Fulcher S, Poehling G. The role of operative arthroscopy for the diagnosis and treatment of lesions about the distal ulna. Hand Clin 1998; 14(2):285–96.

31. Cooney W, Linscheid R, Dobyns J. Triangular fibrocartilage tears. J Hand Surg Am 1994;19(1):143–54.

32. Estrella EP, Hung LK, Ho PC, et al. Arthroscopic repair of triangular fibrocartilage complex tears. Arthroscopy 2007;23(7):729–37, 737. e1.

33. Shih JT, Lee HM, Tan CM. Early isolated triangular fibrocartilage complex tears: management by arthroscopic repair. J Trauma 2002;53(5):922–7.

34. Osterman AL. Arthroscopic Treatment of Radial-Sided TFCC Lesions. International Wrist Investigator's Workshop, ASSH. New York, September 13, 2004.

Arthroscopic Evaluation of the Foveal Attachment of the Triangular Fibrocartilage

David J. Slutsky, MD[a,b],*

KEYWORDS

- Triangular fibrocartilage complex • Arthroscopy
- Foveal attachment • Distal radioulnar joint

RATIONALE

Anatomic and biomechanical studies have highlighted the importance of the deep attachment of the triangular fibrocartilage complex (TFCC) for maintaining stability of the distal radioulnar joint (DRUJ).[1,2] The functional consequence of incompetent foveal fibers is DRUJ instability. Unfortunately there is no accepted standard for DRUJ instability. Berger's definition is that the joint is unstable if it is unable to resist physiologic loads without displacement, with abnormal kinematics throughout the entire arc of motion. (Berger RA, Mayo Clinic Disorders of the Wrist, personal communication, May 2010). He noted that a foveal dislocation will not be fixed by cross-pinning or ulnar shortening. In the absence of a quantifiable objective definition, however, the determination of DRUJ instability is largely dependent on a subjective interpretation of the physical findings.

Although investigators have developed new methods for open reattachment of the foveal attachment,[3,4] arthroscopic repair methods are still in the developmental stage (see the article by Geissler elsewhere in this issue). The standard arthroscopic assessment of the TFCC does not allow one to definitively determine whether the deep fibers are indeed intact, and establishing the diagnosis of a foveal detachment remains an exacting challenge even for the experienced arthroscopist. Ruch and colleagues[5] first described the hook test as a means to test the foveal insertion of the TFCC during the arthroscopic treatment of distal radius fractures whereby if the TFCC can be pulled upwards and radially, this indicates a foveal detachment. Similarly, Tay and colleagues[6] as well as Atzei and colleagues[7] have written that if one can drag the TFCC dorsally with an arthroscopic hook probe, a foveal detachment is indicated. For both methods, however, one must ultimately perform a DRUJ capsulotomy to directly observe the foveal fibers in order to definitively make the diagnosis. Magnetic resonance imaging (MRI) can detect these tears in some instances, but this not only requires a high-power magnet with a dedicated wrist coil and a high-resolution grid with a narrow field of view, but also an experienced musculoskeletal radiologist who can interpret these findings.[8]

RELEVANT ANATOMY
TFCC Anatomy

The TFCC has been well described. It consists of the articular disc, the meniscus homolog, the palmar (PRUL) and dorsal (DRUL) radioulnar ligaments, the extensor carpi ulnaris (ECU), the ulnar capsule, and the ulnolunate and ulnotriquetral ligaments.[9,10] The PRUL and DRUL contain a superficial and a deep portion, which are conjoined at the radius attachment. The superficial portion

[a] Los Angeles County Harbor-UCLA Medical Center, 1000 W. Carson Street, Torrance, CA 90502
[b] The Hand and Wrist Institute, 2808 Columbia Street, Torrance, CA 90503, USA
* The Hand and Wrist Institute, 2808 Columbia Street, Torrance, CA 90503, USA.
E-mail address: d-slutsky@msn.com

Hand Clin 27 (2011) 255–261
doi:10.1016/j.hcl.2011.05.003
0749-0712/11/$ – see front matter

surrounds the articular disc but has no clear definable insertion into the ulnar styloid. The fibers of the deep portion of the DRUL and the PRUL interdigitate to form a conjoined tendon as they converge toward their insertion into the fovea at the base of the ulnar styloid (**Fig. 1**). The foveal insertion has a greater effect on stability than the styloid insertion. Recent work suggests that DRUJ instability may be caused by ulnar detachment.[11] With an intact foveal ligament attachment, patients still may suffer from a peripheral TFCC tear but they may not experience the same instability as those with a total avulsion of the ulnar ligament attachments, which can be seen with an avulsion fracture of the entire ulnar styloid.[12] The ligamentum subcruetum is an inconstant region of vascularized connective tissue that lies between the foveal attachment and the ulnar styloid, but by itself provides little mechanical support.

When examined from a coronal perspective, the ulnar styloid lies relatively dorsal on the end of the ulnar head. The DRUL drapes over the dorsal aspect of the ulnar head as it converges toward the fovea. These factors limit the field of view and make it difficult to insert anything larger than a 1.9-mm scope through a dorsal DRUJ portal. There is more room on the volar ulnar aspect of the DRUJ for insertion of an arthroscope, with relatively unimpeded views of the proximal articular disk and the foveal attachments. The dorsal DRUJ portals remain useful, however, for outflow and for instrumentation (**Fig. 2**).

Dorsal Radioulnar Portals

Both proximal and distal dorsal radioulnar joint portals have been described. These portals lie between the tendons of the ECU and the extensor digiti minimi. In one anatomic study, transverse branches of the dorsal cutaneous branch of the ulnar nerve were the only sensory nerves in proximity to these portals, at a mean of 17.5 mm distally (range 10–20 mm).[13]

Volar Ulnar Portal

In a cadaver study performed by the author, a volar ulnar (VU) portal was established via a 2-cm longitudinal incision made along the ulnar edge of the finger flexor tendons at the proximal wrist crease.[14] The VU portal exploits the same surgical interval as the palmar ulnar approach to the distal radius, which is used in the treatment of displaced articular fractures. The flexor tendons were retracted radially and a trocar was introduced into the radiocarpal joint. The ulnar styloid marked the proximal point of the VU portal, approximately 2 cm distal to the pronator quadratus. The portal was in the same sagittal plane as the ECU subsheath and penetrated the ulnolunate ligament adjacent to the radial insertion of the triangular fibrocartilage (TFC). The ulnar nerve and artery were generally more than 5 mm from the trocar, provided the capsular entry point was deep to the ulnar edge of the profundus tendons. The palmar cutaneous branch of the ulnar nerve (nerve of Henlé) was highly variable and not present in every specimen. This inconstant branch provides sensory fibers to the skin in the distal ulnar and volar part of the forearm to a level 3 cm distal to the wrist crease. Its territory may extend radially beyond the palmaris longus tendon.[15] This branch tends to lie just to the ulnar side of the axis of the

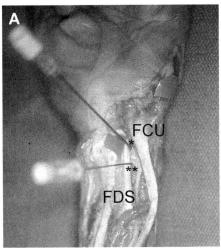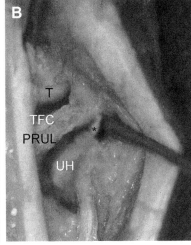

Fig. 1. Volar distal radioulnar (VDRU) portal. (*A*) Relative positions of the volar ulnar (VU) and VDRU portals. FCU, flexor carpi ulnaris; FDS, flexor digitorum sublimus. (*B*) Close-up view of the VDRU portal. Note the foveal attachment of the deep fibers (*asterisk*) of the palmar radioulnar ligament (PRUL). T, triquetrum; UH, ulnar head. (*Courtesy of* David J. Slutsky, MD, Los Angeles, CA.)

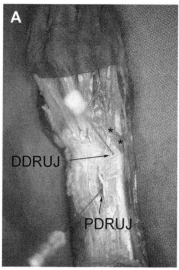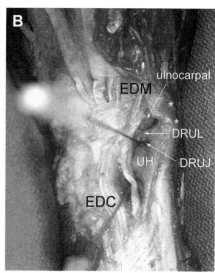

Fig. 2. Dorsal DRUJ portals. (*A*) Relative positions of the proximal (PDRUJ) and distal (DDRUJ) portals in relation to the dorsal cutaneous branch of the ulnar nerve (*asterisk*). (*B*) Close-up view of the portals with a needle in the ulnocarpal joint and dorsal DRUJ. DRUL, dorsal radioulnar ligament; ECU, extensor carpi ulnaris; EDM, extensor digiti minimi; UH, ulnar head. (*Courtesy of* David J. Slutsky, MD, Los Angeles, CA.)

fourth ray, but it was absent in 43% of specimens in one study.[16] Martin and colleagues[17] demonstrated that there was no true internervous plane because of the presence of multiple ulnar-based cutaneous nerves to the palm, which puts them at risk with any ulnar incision. Because there is no true safe zone, careful dissection and wound-spread technique should be observed.

PHYSICAL EXAMINATION

An assessment is made of the amount of DRUJ instability by manually translating the radius dorsal and palmar to the distal ulna as well as its "end point," and compared with the opposite side in full pronation, supination, and in neutral. This assessment should also be done in 30° of pronation because the deep fibers are not used in this position, hence only the superficial volar and dorsal radioulnar ligaments are tested. The foveal fibers may also be assessed by gauging the amount of translation in neutral and then the test repeated with the wrist in ulnar deviation (Tommy Lindau, personal communication, 2009). The ulnar head should be checked for a positive piano-key sign. With the wrist in pronation, the unstable distal ulna may translate dorsally and can be manually reduced with dorsal thumb pressure, similar to depressing a piano key.[18] Jupiter[19] has noted that it is difficult to quantify distal radioulnar instability, and that these methods suffer from subjectivity and lack of interobserver validity. Moreover,

it is a static versus a dynamic assessment of the stability associated with forearm rotation. In the setting of an acute unstable distal radius fracture, he opined that the surgeon should compress the ulna to the radius after plate fixation and then rotate the hand and wrist. A palpable clunk would suggest true instability and might indicate a disruption of the distal oblique band of the interosseous membrane, as described by Noda and colleagues.[20]

INDICATIONS FOR DRUJ ARTHROSCOPY

An arthroscopic assessment of the distal radioulnar joint is indicated in any patient with acute or chronic DRUJ instability that is suspected by either physical examination, dorsal or palmar translation of the ulnar head on a true lateral radiographic view (ie, with the scaphoid, lunate, and triquetrum superimposed),[21] or an axial computed tomographic view.[22] It is also useful in cases of a symptomatic and displaced basilar ulnar styloid nonunion where one must decide whether to simply resect the ulnar styloid or to perform an open reduction and internal fixation of the styloid rather than a styloid excision and foveal reattachment.

CONTRAINDICATIONS

Absolute contraindications would include infection, neurovascular injury, or a poor soft-tissue envelope. Relative contraindications would include massive edema and/or a distortion of the anatomy, such as seen with a distal radius fracture or carpal dislocation whereby the ulnar neurovascular bundle is at increased risk for injury.

SURGICAL TECHNIQUE OF DRUJ ARTHROSCOPY

The VU portal is established via a 2-cm longitudinal incision centered over the proximal wrist crease along the ulnar edge of the finger flexor. The tendons are retracted to the radial side and the radiocarpal joint space is identified with a 22-gauge needle. Blunt tenotomy scissors or forceps are used to pierce the volar capsule, followed by insertion of a cannula and blunt trocar, then the arthroscope. Care is taken to situate the cannula beneath the ulnar edge of the flexor tendons and to apply retraction in a radial direction alone, in order to avoid injury to the ulnar nerve and artery. The median nerve is protected by the interposed flexor tendons. The palmar region of the lunotriquetral interosseous ligament can usually be seen slightly distal and radial to the portal. A hook probe is inserted through the 6-R or 6-U portal.

Volar Distal Radioulnar Portal

The topographic landmarks and establishment of the volar distal radioulnar (VDRU) portal are identical to those of the VU portal. The capsular entry point lies 5 to 10 mm proximally.[23]

The VDRU portal is accessed through the VU skin incision. A 1.9-mm joint arthroscope can be used because gaining access to the DRUJ can be difficult, especially in a small wrist, but the author has found that a standard 2.7-mm scope provides a better field of view. The ulnocarpal joint

is first identified as already described. It is useful to leave a needle or cannula in the ulnocarpal joint for reference during this step. The DRUJ is then located by angling a 22-gauge needle 45° proximally, then injecting the DRUJ with saline. Alternatively, the skin incision can be extended proximally for 1 cm so that it lies at the same level as the VDRU capsular entry point. Once the correct plane is identified, the volar DRUJ capsule is pierced with tenotomy scissors followed by a cannula with a blunt trocar and then the arthroscope. Alternatively, a probe can be placed in the distal dorsal radioulnar joint portal and advanced through the palmar incision to help locate the joint space. It can then be used as a switching stick over which the cannula is introduced. Initially, the DRUJ space appears quite confined, but over the course of 3 to 5 minutes the fluid irrigation expands the joint space, which improves visibility (**Fig. 3**). A burr or thermal probe can be substituted for the 3-mm hook probe through the dorsal DRUJ portal as necessary.

Dorsal DRUJ Portals

The dorsal radioulnar joint can be accessed through a proximal and distal portal.[24] The proximal portal (PDRUJ) is located in the axilla of the joint, just proximal to the sigmoid notch and the flare of the ulnar metaphysis. This portal is easier to penetrate and should be used initially to prevent chondral injury from insertion of the trocar. The forearm is held in supination to relax the dorsal capsule and to move the ulnar head volarly. This maneuver also lifts the central disk distally from the head of the ulna. Reducing the traction to 1 to 2 lb (0.45–0.9 kg) permits better views between the ulna and the sigmoid notch by reducing the

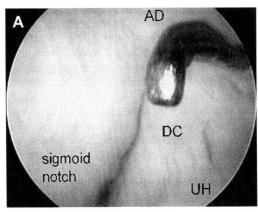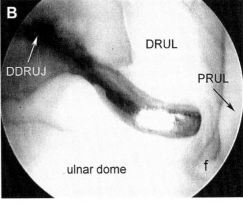

Fig. 3. View from the VDRU portal. (*A*) The proximal sigmoid notch is well visualized. The dorsal DRUJ capsule (DC) can be seen arising from the ulnar head (UH). The probe is in the dorsal, distal DRUJ portal. AD, articular disc. (*B*) Moving the scope distally and ulnarly, the dorsal radioulnar ligament (DRUL) and the palmar radioulnar ligament (PRUL) can be seen inserting on the fovea (f). DDRUJ, dorsal DRUJ portal. (*Courtesy of* David J. Slutsky, MD, Los Angeles, CA.)

compressive force caused by axial traction. The joint space is identified by first inserting a 22-gauge needle horizontally at the neck of the distal ulna. Fluoroscopy facilitates the needle placement. The joint is infiltrated with saline and the capsule is spread with tenotomy scissors through a small incision. A small cannula and trocar for the 1.9-mm scope are introduced, followed by insertion of a 1.9-mm 30° angle scope. Entry into this portal provides views of the proximal sigmoid notch cartilage and the articular surface of the neck of the ulna. One should systematically look for loose bodies or synovial hypertrophy.

The distal portal (DDRUJ) is identified 6 to 8 mm distally with the 22-gauge needle and just proximal to the 6-R portal. This portal can be used for outflow drainage or for instrumentation. It lies on top of the ulnar head but underneath the TFC, hence it cannot be used in the presence of a positive ulnar variance. The TFC has the least tension

in neutral rotation of the forearm, which is the optimal position for visualizing the articular dome of the ulnar head, the undersurface of the TFC, and the foveal insertion of the PRUL. Because of the dorsal entry of the arthroscope, the course of the DRUL is not visible until its attachment into the fovea is encountered.[25]

Atzei and colleagues[7] have described a direct foveal portal. This portal is 1 cm proximal to the 6-U portal (**Fig. 4**). The scope is inserted with the wrist in full supination because the ulnar styloid and the ECU tendon displace dorsally, and the fovea and the ulnar-most area of the distal ulna become subcutaneous.

COMPLICATIONS

The most feared complication from this approach would be an injury to the ulnar neurovascular bundle or the finger flexor tendons due to the

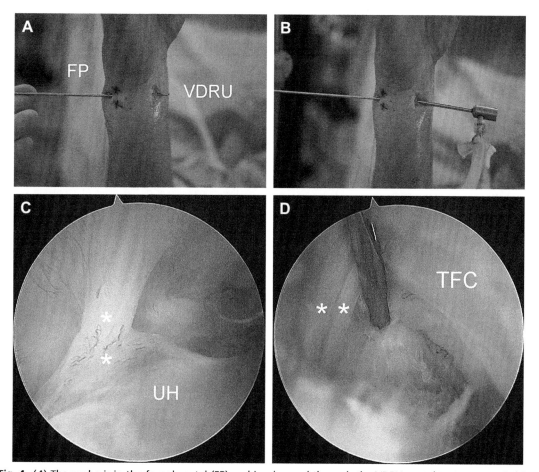

Fig. 4. (*A*) The probe is in the foveal portal (FP) and is advanced through the VDRU portal to act as a switching stick. (*B*) The cannula is advanced over the probe and into the distal radioulnar joint. (*C*) View of the foveal fibers (*asterisks*) from the VDRU attaching to the ulnar head (UH). (*D*) The needle is placed through the foveal portal and used to tension the foveal fibers (*asterisks*). TFC, triangular fibrocartilage. (*Courtesy of* David J. Slutsky, MD, Los Angeles, CA.)

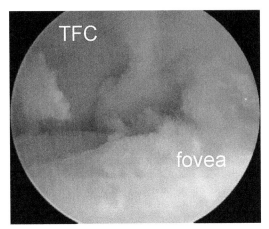

Fig. 5. Foveal tear. View from the VDRU demonstrating a bare foveal area. TFC, triangular fibrocartilage. (*Courtesy of* David J. Slutsky, MD, Los Angeles, CA.)

surgical approach when developing the VU portal. Chondral injury to the ulnar head is possible as well as iatrogenic injury to the foveal ligaments or volar radioulnar ligament. None of these complications were encountered in the author's series.

RESULTS

The VU portal has been used in 68 patients since 1998. The volar aspect of the DRUJ was accessed in 14 of these patients to rule out a tear of the deep foveal attachment of the TFCC. A preoperative MRI in each patient could not definitively determine whether the foveal fibers were indeed intact. The foveal attachment of the TFC was seen to be intact in 8 of 14 patients, and directly contributed to the decision made as to the type of surgical treatment. In 2 patients the attachment was poorly seen, due to foveal scarring from an associated peripheral TFCC tear, and the DRUJ portal was not helpful. In 2 cases the TFCC and the foveal fibers were intact but the radioulnar ligaments were attenuated. These patients were treated with an open dorsal radioulnar imbrication and a tendon graft reconstruction of the DRUJ, as described by Adams and Berger.[26] In 2 patients the foveal fibers were clearly torn (**Fig. 5**). These patients were treated with a tendon graft reconstruction of the DRUJ and a foveal repair of the TFCC.

REFERENCES

1. Hagert CG. The distal radioulnar joint in relation to the whole forearm. Clin Orthop Relat Res 1992; 275:56–64.
2. Schuind F, An KN, Berglund L, et al. The distal radio-ulnar ligaments: a biomechanical study. J Hand Surg Am 1991;16:1106–14.
3. Moritomo H. Advantages of open repair of a foveal tear of the triangular fibrocartilage complex via a palmar surgical approach. Tech Hand Up Extrem Surg 2009;13:176–81.
4. Nakamura T, Nakao Y, Ikegami H, et al. Open repair of the ulnar disruption of the triangular fibrocartilage complex with double three-dimensional mattress suturing technique. Tech Hand Up Extrem Surg 2004;8:116–23.
5. Ruch DS, Yang CC, Smith BP. Results of acute arthroscopically repaired triangular fibrocartilage complex injuries associated with intra-articular distal radius fractures. Arthroscopy 2003;19:511–6.
6. Tay SC, Tomita K, Berger RA. The "ulnar fovea sign" for defining ulnar wrist pain: an analysis of sensitivity and specificity. J Hand Surg Am 2007;32:438–44.
7. Atzei A, Rizzo A, Luchetti R, et al. Arthroscopic foveal repair of triangular fibrocartilage complex peripheral lesion with distal radioulnar joint instability. Tech Hand Up Extrem Surg 2008;12:226–35.
8. Amrami KK, Felmlee JP. 3-Tesla imaging of the wrist and hand: techniques and applications. Semin Musculoskelet Radiol 2008;12:223–37.
9. Palmer AK, Werner FW. The triangular fibrocartilage complex of the wrist—anatomy and function. J Hand Surg Am 1981;6:153–62.
10. Ishii S, Palmer AK, Werner FW, et al. An anatomic study of the ligamentous structure of the triangular fibrocartilage complex. J Hand Surg Am 1998;23:977–85.
11. Adams BD, Samani JE, Holley KA. Triangular fibrocartilage injury: a laboratory model. J Hand Surg Am 1996;21:189–93.
12. Haugstvedt JR, Berger RA, Nakamura T, et al. Relative contributions of the ulnar attachments of the triangular fibrocartilage complex to the dynamic stability of the distal radioulnar joint. J Hand Surg Am 2006;31:445–51.
13. Abrams RA, Petersen M, Botte MJ. Arthroscopic portals of the wrist: an anatomic study. J Hand Surg Am 1994;19:940–4.
14. Slutsky DJ. The use of a volar ulnar portal in wrist arthroscopy. Arthroscopy 2004;20:158–63.
15. Balogh B, Valencak J, Vesely M, et al. The nerve of Henle: an anatomic and immunohistochemical study. J Hand Surg Am 1999;24:1103–8.
16. McCabe SJ, Kleinert JM. The nerve of Henle. J Hand Surg Am 1990;15:784–8.
17. Martin CH, Seiler JG 3rd, Lesesne JS. The cutaneous innervation of the palm: an anatomic study of the ulnar and median nerves. J Hand Surg Am 1996;21:634–8.
18. Szabo RM. Distal radioulnar joint instability. J Bone Joint Surg Am 2006;88:884–94.
19. Jupiter JB. Commentary: the effect of ulnar styloid fractures on patient-rated outcomes after volar locking plating of distal radius fractures. J Hand Surg Am 2009;34:1603–4.

20. Noda K, Goto A, Murase T, et al. Interosseous membrane of the forearm: an anatomical study of ligament attachment locations. J Hand Surg Am 2009;34:415–22.
21. Mino DE, Palmer AK, Levinsohn EM. Radiography and computerized tomography in the diagnosis of incongruity of the distal radio-ulnar joint. A prospective study. J Bone Joint Surg Am 1985;67:247–52.
22. Kim JP, Park MJ. Assessment of distal radioulnar joint instability after distal radius fracture: comparison of computed tomography and clinical examination results. J Hand Surg Am 2008;33:1486–92.
23. Slutsky DJ. Distal radioulnar joint arthroscopy and the volar ulnar portal. Tech Hand Up Extrem Surg 2007;11:38–44.
24. Whipple TL. Arthroscopy of the distal radioulnar joint. Indications, portals, and anatomy. Hand Clin 1994;10:589–92.
25. Berger RA. Arthroscopic anatomy of the wrist and distal radioulnar joint. Hand Clin 1999;15:393–413, vii.
26. Adams BD, Berger RA. An anatomic reconstruction of the distal radioulnar ligaments for posttraumatic distal radioulnar joint instability. J Hand Surg Am 2002;27:243–51.

Foveal TFCC Tear Classification and Treatment

Andrea Atzei, MD[a,b,c,*], Riccardo Luchetti, MD[d,e]

KEYWORDS

- Triangular fibrocartilage complex • Foveal tear
- Arthroscopy • Treatment algorithm • DRUJ instability

Disorders of the triangular fibrocartilage complex (TFCC) represent one of the most frequent causes of ulnar-sided pain and disability in the wrist. TFCC lesions are currently categorized according to the classification system proposed by Andrew K. Palmer[1] in 1989, which considers two main classes: Class 1, Traumatic lesions and Class 2, Degenerative lesions. These classes are further divided into different types, depending on the location of the tear and the presence or absence of associated chondromalacic changes. Class 1 traumatic lesions are organized according to the tear's location. Type 1-B injuries consist of traumatic tears involving the ulnar periphery of the TFCC and may be associated with an ulnar styloid fracture. Histologic and functional anatomy show that the ulnar side of the TFCC is arranged in a complex tridimensional structure and consists of 3 components: the proximal triangular ligament, the distal hammock structure, and the ulnar collateral ligament (UCL).[2]

According to its structure and function, the UCL is assimilated to the distal hammock structure to make up the distal component of the TFCC (dc-TFCC), which supports and suspends the ulnar carpus.[2] The proximal component of the TFCC (pc-TFCC) is represented by the proximal triangular ligament and consists of the strong ligamentous structure that stabilizes the distal radioulnar joint (DRUJ). It is also described as "ligamentum subcruentum,"[3] and is made up of the DRUJ ligaments, palmar and dorsal, whose ulnar insertion is located in the fovea rather than in the ulnar styloid (**Fig. 1**).

The fovea ulnaris represents the "convergent point" of insertion for the pc-TFCC and for the fibers of the palmar ulnocarpal ligaments.[4] Hence the foveal insertion of the TFCC plays a key role in the stability of both the DRUJ and the ulnocarpal joint.

Type 1-B TFCC tears may occur following a violent traction and twisting of the wrist or forearm or, more commonly, a fall on the outstretched hand, which may also cause a fracture of the distal radius. According to the magnitude and direction of the traumatic force acting on the ulnar wrist, the TFCC components may tear in a variable manner. When there is an isolated rupture of the dc-TFCC, DRUJ stability is preserved. However, when a Type 1-B TFCC tear involves disruption of the pc-TFCC the DRUJ becomes unstable, leading to ulnar-sided pain, reduced grip strength, decreased forearm rotation, and clinical signs of DRUJ instability. When overlooked, DRUJ instability may be a cause of an unsatisfactory result and require reoperation. Estrella and colleagues[5] reviewed the clinical and functional outcomes of 35 patients treated by arthroscopic repair of TFCC tears and found that of the 26% of patients with an unsatisfactory result, 45% of these were related to persistent DRUJ instability.

a Hand Surgery and Rehabilitation Team, Viale della Repubblica 10/B, 31050 Villorba (TV), Italy
b Policlinico "San Giorgio", Via Gemelli 10, 33170 Pordenone, Italy
c Department of Orthopaedic Surgery, Azienda Ospedaliera-Universitaria, Verona, Italy
d Rimini Hand Center, Via Pietro da Rimini 4, 47900 Rimini, Italy
e Department of Hand Surgery, Clinic of Plastic and Reconstructive Surgery, Multimedica Milano, Via Milanese 300, 20138 Milano, Italy
* Corresponding author.
E-mail address: andreatzei@libero.it

Hand Clin 27 (2011) 263–272
doi:10.1016/j.hcl.2011.05.014

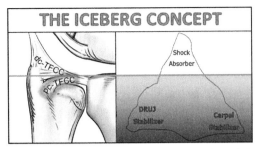

THE ICEBERG CONCEPT

Shock Absorber

dc-TFCC
pc-TFCC

DRUJ Stabilizer   Carpal Stabilizer

Fig. 1. Artist's rendering of the ulnar portion of the TFCC. It is separated into the distal component (dc-TFCC) formed by the UCL and the distal hammock structure, and the proximal component (pc-TFCC), represented by the proximal triangular ligament, or ligamentum subcruentum, which originates from the ulnar fovea and the proximal styloid and stabilizes the DRUJ. The "iceberg" concept, with an immediate visual representation, summarizes TFCC functions, its importance, and difficulty of assessment from simple observation of the emerging part (as in radiocarpal arthroscopy).

Anderson and colleagues,[6] comparing the clinical results of arthroscopic (36 patients) and open (39 patients) repair of traumatic TFCC tears, found a 26.6% rate of reoperation, without any statistically significant difference between the two groups. These investigators also found that 65% of the reoperations were required to address DRUJ instability, and related this finding to either failure to diagnose true DRUJ instability or an inadequate TFCC repair. Thus the controversy about the value of the arthroscopic repair method as compared with an open transosseous repair of peripheral tears[3,7–9] is still unsolved, because it is currently assumed that only the latter method can restore the foveal insertion of the TFCC in the case of DRUJ instability.[3]

IMPROVING UNDERSTANDING OF TFCC PERIPHERAL TEARS: THE ICEBERG CONCEPT

During the last two decades an increased knowledge of functional anatomy and pathophysiology of the TFCC, along with technical refinements in the arthroscopic and surgical repair of the TFCC, have contributed to a dramatic change of the surgeons' perspective toward the TFCC. The earlier concept of the TFCC as the "hammock" structure of the ulnar carpus has been reconsidered and updated to the novel "iceberg" concept (see **Fig. 1**). In analogy with the iceberg, during arthroscopy of the radiocarpal joint (RCJ) the TFCC shows its "emerging" tip. The tip of the iceberg represents that part of the TFCC that functions as a shock absorber. It is of reduced size compared with the "submerged" part, which can

be seen only through distal radioulnar (DRU) arthroscopy. The submerged TFCC represents the foveal insertions of the TFCC and functions as the stabilizer of the DRUJ and of the ulnar carpus. The larger size of the submerged portion of the iceberg corresponds to its greater functional importance.

This change of perspective went together with the growing need for a revised approach to the peripheral TFCC tear[5,10] that can provide a more accurate definition of the spectrum of different tears, in order to provide reliable guidelines for surgical indications and allow an improved comparison of different surgical techniques.

According to the authors' personal experience, this article presents an algorithm of the treatment of traumatic peripheral TFCC tear based on clinical, radiological, and arthroscopic findings.

CLINICAL ASSESSMENT

On a systematic examination of the painful wrist, the differential diagnosis and/or confirmation of the diagnosis of a peripheral TFCC tear is achieved by means of special provocative maneuvers and diagnostic tests.[3,11] The most reliable clinical sign of a peripheral TFCC tear is the ulnar fovea sign,[12] whereby the patient has point tenderness over the ulnar capsule just palmar to the extensor carpi ulnaris (ECU) tendon (**Fig. 2**). Pain is exacerbated by passive forearm rotation and may be associated with the presence of a "click" or "crepitus," or an intra-articular grinding sensation. Resisted rotational movements are often weak and reproduce the patient's complaints.

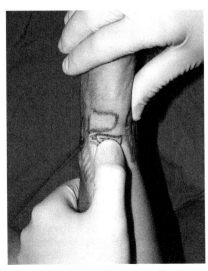

Fig. 2. The fovea sign elicits pain in the dotted area between extensor carpi ulnaris (ECU) and flexor carpi ulnaris (FCU). It is positive for a peripheral TFCC laceration.

A simple and reliable test to assess DRUJ laxity is the ballottement test.[13] This test consists of passive anteroposterior and posteroanterior translation of the ulna on the radius in neutral rotation, in full supination and pronation. Abnormal translation of the ulnar head suggests a complete TFCC disruption (**Fig. 3**). The test is repeated with the forearm in full supination and pronation, in an attempt to understand which limb of the DRUJ ligament is ruptured, either the dorsal or the palmar DRUJ, respectively. The authors recommend the evaluation of the resistance at the end point of the translation. This finding is of utmost importance because the amount of DRUJ laxity correlates with the clinical DRUJ instability. Although there may be increased laxity, the DRUJ that demonstrates a "firm" end point is unlikely to progress toward a clinically symptomatic instability. Conversely, the DRUJ showing an increased passive anteroposterior or posteroanterior laxity with a "soft" end point is prone to develop a clinical

instability, that is, cause a patient's complaint when left untreated.

Provided the forearm muscles are relaxed, provocative maneuvers for DRUJ instability may show greater laxity of the painful wrist as compared with the opposite side. Protective contraction of the muscular stabilizers, especially the ECU and the pronator quadratus of the DRUJ, may mislead the surgeon with false-negative findings. Because of this, it is recommended that the DRUJ stability should be retested when the patient is under regional anesthesia before the operation. In the acute setting, that is, when there is the suspicion of a TFCC tear associated with an intra-articular or extra-articular distal radius fracture, it is strongly recommended that the ballottement test be assessed intraoperatively after reduction and stable fixation of the fracture.

IMAGING ASSESSMENT

All patients presenting with acute or chronic wrist pain should have radiographs taken of the wrist. Usually these are of limited value for diagnosing isolated TFCC tears, but evidence of distal ulna displacement, the presence of DRUJ widening, or/and ulnar styloid fracture may give a hint of an associated DRUJ instability.

The presence of an ulnar styloid fracture is no longer considered an absolute indicator of DRUJ instability, but only as a risk factor,[14–16] regardless of the fragment size and displacement. The supposition by Hauck[17] that DRUJ is unstable when the styloid is fractured at the base, and the opposite when the fracture is at the tip, has not been confirmed in several arthroscopic studies,[14,18–20] which did not find any predictable correlation between an ulnar styloid fractures and a TFCC tear. Although the ulnar styloid fracture is related to the pattern and magnitude of the injury sustained, it also depends on the bone quality and the relative strength of the ligaments. Thus an ulnar styloid fracture is more common in cases of osteoporotic bone, which may explain the scarcity of isolated ligamentous injury in the elderly as compared with young active patients, in whom DRUJ instability often results from a midsubstance tear of the TFCC.[21]

When the TFCC tear is associated with a distal radius fracture, it should be evaluated and eventually repaired at the time of fracture fixation, after the fracture realignment. Likewise, when a TFCC tear is associated with a malunited extra-articular fracture of the radius and/or ulna, it is advisable to reduce any angulation, shortening, and/or translation of the malunited fragment with a corrective osteotomy before any TFCC repair or reconstruction.

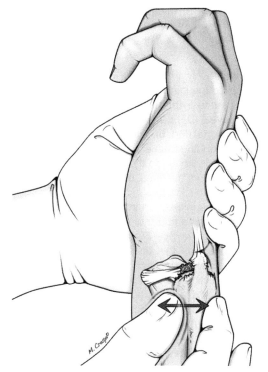

Fig. 3. The ballottement test evaluates DRUJ stability. The radius is grasped by the examiner and the distal ulna, fixed between the examiner's thumb and index finger, and moved in dorsal and palmar directions with respect to the radius. If the ulna shows an increased displacement relative to the contralateral side associated with a "soft" end-point resistance, it is likely to develop a symptomatic DRUJ instability, that is, it may be a cause of pain when left untreated.

The Galeazzi fracture-subluxation is a particular condition that is frequently associated with a TFCC tear. When the fracture is located within 7.5 cm of the distal epiphysis of the radius, DRUJ instability is a common finding even after proper fracture reduction, and may require[22] a TFCC reattachment to the ulna, although forearm immobilization in full supination for 8 weeks may also suffice.

Yet another controversial issue concerns the usefulness of magnetic resonance imaging (MRI) in the diagnosis of a peripheral TFCC tear. Whereas an MRI arthrogram may be both sensitive and specific in diagnosing a tear, it has not shown similar accuracy in assessing the tear size and location,[23] and eventually the quality of the tear's edges and its healing potential. Studies comparing specificity and sensitivity of arthrography, MRI, and arthroscopy confirm arthroscopic visualization of a TFCC tear to be the gold standard for definitive diagnosis.[24,25] However, MRI may be useful to exclude associated pathologies of the ulnar compartment.

ARTHROSCOPIC ASSESSMENT

Accurate classification of the different conditions affecting the TFCC requires evaluation of both the distal and proximal component of the TFCC, which should be done by radiocarpal and DRU arthroscopy, respectively.

Radiocarpal arthroscopy permits one to evaluate the dc-TFCC. With the scope in the standard 3–4 portal, the tear is visualized in the dorsoulnar corner of the TFCC and probed through the 6-R portal. As a rule TFCC tension is assessed by the trampoline test,[8] which evaluates the TFCC resilience ("trampoline effect") by applying a compressive load across it with the probe. The test is positive when the TFCC is soft and compliant, usually due to a tear at its periphery (**Fig. 4**).

To achieve a specific assessment of the foveal insertion of the proximal component of the TFCC, the hook test has been recently proposed.[10,26,27] The hook test consists of applying traction to the ulnar-most border of the TFCC with the probe inserted through the 4–5 or 6-R portal, and is considered positive when the TFCC can be displaced toward the center of the radiocarpal joint (**Fig. 5**). DRU arthroscopy is the only method to directly visualize any ligamentous tear of the pc-TFCC or avulsion from the fovea. As the DRUJ is a very narrow and tight joint, occasionally DRU arthroscopy is difficult to perform in the healthy joint, when the pc-TFCC is still intact. However, when the pc-TFCC is torn, the articular disk is loose and more space is available for DRUJ exploration. An 18-gauge hypodermic needle may be placed

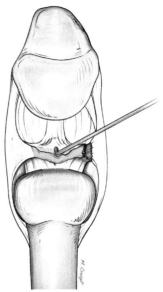

Fig. 4. The trampoline test. The probe inserted through 6-R (or 4–5) portal applies a pressure across the TFCC and shows a lack of the normal resilience when the TFCC is lacerated. This test may be misleading when using the dry technique, probably due to the lack of fluid distention that reduces TFCC resilience.

percutaneously through the dorsal DRUJ portals to localize the joint. A more accurate assessment can be made by probing the pc-TFCC through the direct foveal (DF) portal, located 1 cm proximal to the 6-U portal (**Fig. 6**). The DF portal is less technically demanding than establishing a volar portal,[28] but its use is limited to the introduction of working instruments in the area of the ulnar styloid and fovea.

The probe is inserted into the joint close to the fovea to lift the articular disk and palpate the foveal insertion of the pc-TFCC. In the authors' early experience with this test, DRU arthroscopy was used routinely to inspect the proximal TFCC, and showed a high correlation between the positive hook test and a disruption of TFCC foveal insertion. In the authors' practice a positive hook test is a consistent indicator of a TFCC foveal avulsion, and confirmatory DRU arthroscopy is no longer considered necessary. However, DRU arthroscopy is still advisable to detect any posttraumatic chondromalacia or even cartilage loss of the distal ulna or sigmoid notch that may be the cause of a poor outcome after TFCC foveal repair.[10]

Radiocarpal and DRU arthroscopy provide a combination of findings that should be considered when deciding on the appropriate treatment for a TFCC tear. These findings are summarized by the following classes.

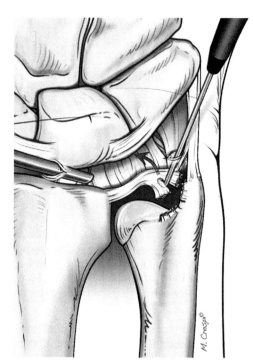

Fig. 5. The hook test. The probe is inserted through the 6-R portal into the prestyloid recess in an attempt to pull the TFCC in multiple directions. The TFCC can be displaced toward the center of the radiocarpal joint only when the proximal component of the TFCC is torn or avulsed from the fovea. In this case the test is considered positive.

Lacerated Components of the Triangular Fibrocartilage Complex

Establishing the extent of TFCC peripheral tear is of outmost importance, because each component, namely dc-TFCC and pc-TFCC, may be involved either separately or in association.

Therefore 3 different types of lesion are possible:

1. *Distal tear (isolated tear of the distal component of the TFCC).* When only the dc-TFCC is lacerated, the trampoline test is positive for loss of TFCC resilience, but the hook test is negative. The Integrity of pc-TFCC insertion onto the ulna may be confirmed by DRU arthroscopy.
2. *Complete tear (tear of both distal and proximal component of the TFCC).* A Complete peripheral TFCC tear involves both components of the TFCC. A tear of the dc-TFCC is visible during radiocarpal arthroscopy, and pc-TFCC avulsion may be demonstrated by DRU arthroscopy. Both trampoline and hook tests are positive.
3. *Proximal tear (isolated tear of the proximal component of the TFCC).* Standard radiocarpal arthroscopy fails to show any abnormalities of the TFCC's peripheral contour and capsular reflection. However, both trampoline and hook tests are positive. The tear involves a laceration of only the pc-TFCC or avulsion from the fovea ulnaris. It can be confirmed by DRU arthroscopy (**Fig. 7**).

Understanding which TFCC component is lacerated leads to an appropriate treatment modality. In

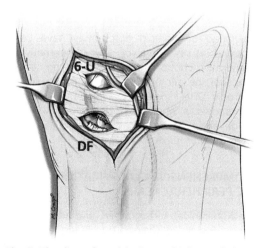

Fig. 6. The direct foveal (DF) portal is located about 1 cm proximal to the 6-U portal and allows exposure of the basi-styloid and foveal area. It can also be prepared as a mini open approach through an oblique skin incision between the ECU and FCU tendons, protection of the dorsal branch of the ulnar nerve, and splitting of the extensor retinaculum.

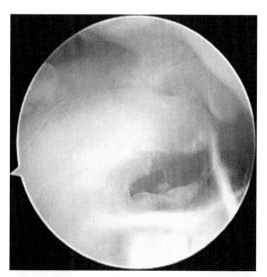

Fig. 7. In Class 2 and 3 TFCC peripheral tears, the hook test is positive and DRU arthroscopy confirms the laceration of the proximal TFCC close to its foveal insertions.

the case of a proximal or complete tear, TFCC reinsertion onto the fovea ulnaris is recommended. However, in cases of a distal tear, arthroscopic suturing of the TFCC to the dorsal ulnocarpal joint capsule and the ECU tendon subsheath is appropriate.

Reparability of the Triangular Fibrocartilage Complex Tear

When there is a small TFCC tear, as well as in the case of an avulsion type of rupture, the tear's edges can be reapproximated or reduced easily and the TFCC repair can be performed with success. By contrast, in the presence of a massive rupture of the TFCC and/or retraction of the ligamentous remnants (**Fig. 8**), proper tear closure or reapproximation of the avulsed ligament to its anatomic position is not feasible. Furthermore, chronic midsubstance ligamentous tears may show degenerated or necrotic edges that are difficult to debride with the shaver to a well-vascularized area. A repair is unlikely to provide adequate healing. The same applies for the elongated and frayed ligament following a failed suture: direct repair is unlikely to be successful, and TFCC reconstruction with a tendon graft is recommended (**Fig. 9**). In the authors' experience, a pc-TFCC tear has a good healing potential for up to 3 months after injury (acute tears), whereas tears treated from 3 to 6 months after injury (subacute tears) have unpredictable characteristics, and more chronic tears usually have a poor healing potential. Moreover, ligamentous disorders (eg, chondrocalcinosis) or congenital dysmorphisms of the styloid and foveal

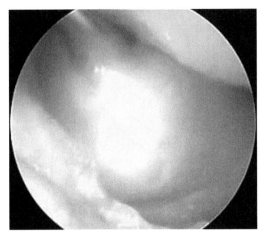

Fig. 9. Class 4-B nonrepairable peripheral TFCC tear as seen through radiocarpal arthroscopy. The probe is elevating a very thin and atrophic TFCC, which is not amenable to repair.

area of the ulna (eg, styloid hypoplasia, flattened ulnar head) represent further conditions that are associated with a poor healing potential after repair (**Fig. 10**).

When direct repair is likely to fail because of the aforementioned conditions, reconstruction with a tendon graft should be taken into consideration.[29,30]

Cartilage Status of the Distal Radioulnar Joint

Well-preserved cartilage is the prerequisite of utmost importance when planning any repair or reconstruction for a TFCC disruption. Following high-energy trauma, a cartilage defect over the ulnar head or sigmoid notch may have been produced at the time of injury. Alternatively, degenerative chondromalacia may be the consequence of the altered joint kinematics, resulting in chronic DRUJ instability. When DRU arthroscopy shows a chondral defect in the DRUJ, salvage arthroplasty techniques are recommended as an alternative.[31–36]

A COMPREHENSIVE CLASSIFICATION OF TFCC PERIPHERAL TEARS

Based on clinical, radiographic, and arthroscopic findings, 6 classes (Classes 0 to 5) are defined in a comprehensive classification that considers the different types of peripheral TFCC lesions and the ulnar styloid. Each class is provided with guidelines for specific treatment modalities: suture repair, foveal refixation, reconstruction with tendon graft, or salvage procedures (arthroplasty or joint replacement) (**Fig. 11**).

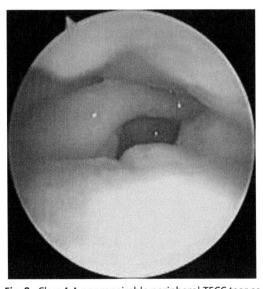

Fig. 8. Class 4-A nonrepairable peripheral TFCC tear as seen through radiocarpal arthroscopy. Note the large gap between the rounded sclerotic tear's edges.

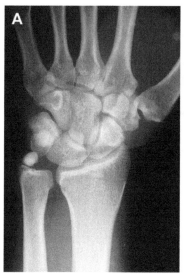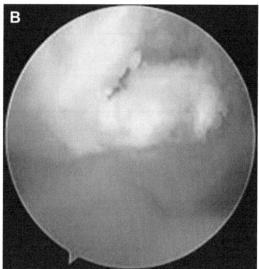

Fig. 10. Nonrepairable peripheral TFCC tear due to chondrocalcinosis of the DRUJ. (*A*) Plain radiograph shows a slightly widened DRUJ and an area of calcium deposit close to the fovea ulnaris. Ballottement test confirms DRUJ laxity with a soft end-point resistance. (*B*) DRU arthroscopy shows the calcium deposit within the degenerated fibers of the proximal TFCC.

Clinical assessment by the ballottement test permits evaluation of DRUJ instability as: Negative (Stable DRUJ); Hyperlax joint/Slight instability (increased translation with hard end point); Mild to Severe instability (increased translation with soft end point).

Plain radiographs of the wrist are taken to confirm correct alignment of the distal radius and ulna and to reveal any fracture of the ulnar styloid. Two conditions are defined: when the styloid is intact or shows a fracture at the tip and when the styloid fracture is close to its base (basilar fracture).

Radiocarpal arthroscopy is used to reveal a laceration of the TFCC along its peripheral margin and to evaluate the tear's size and the quality of TFCC remnants to determine the feasibility of repair. The arthroscopic hook test is used to assess proper tautness of the proximal insertion of the TFCC. When the TFCC is taut (negative hook test) the proximal foveal insertion of the TFCC is preserved. However, the presence of a loose TFCC (positive hook test) is suggestive of a disruption of the TFCC foveal insertion, due to either ligamentous tearing or avulsion with a basilar fracture of the ulnar styloid. DRU arthroscopy allows for an evaluation of the DRUJ cartilage to assess any cartilage defect that contraindicates repair or reconstruction.

AN ALGORITHM OF TREATMENT

The most common clinical conditions involving traumatic TFCC peripheral tear are summarized according to the aforementioned classes with the

intention of providing a foundation for the therapeutic algorithm.

Class 0: Isolated Styloid Fracture Without TFCC Tear

An ulnar styloid fracture is present as an isolated finding. This condition is frequently associated with a distal radius fracture, especially in the elderly. Arthroscopy, which may be performed for the assisted reduction of the radius fracture, shows a normal TFCC appearance. The DRUJ is clinically stable. Acute cases require wrist splinting for pain relief for about 3 weeks. When there is an associated distal radius fracture, the patients are treated according to the rehabilitation protocol for a distal radius fracture. Patients may seldom develop chronic pain due to a persistent ulnar styloid nonunion or ulnar styloid impaction syndrome,[37] and require fragment removal.

Class 1: Distal Peripheral TFCC Tear

A peripheral tear of the TFCC involves an isolated laceration of the distal component, which may be associated with an ulnar styloid fracture. The DRUJ may be slightly lax, but the ballottement test demonstrates a hard end point. Radiocarpal arthroscopy shows a distal peripheral tear, and the hook test is negative for a proximal TFCC disruption. DRUJ cartilage is unaffected. Healing of a small tear usually requires at least 4 weeks of wrist immobilization, followed by 2 weeks in which splinting is weaned. A larger tear requires

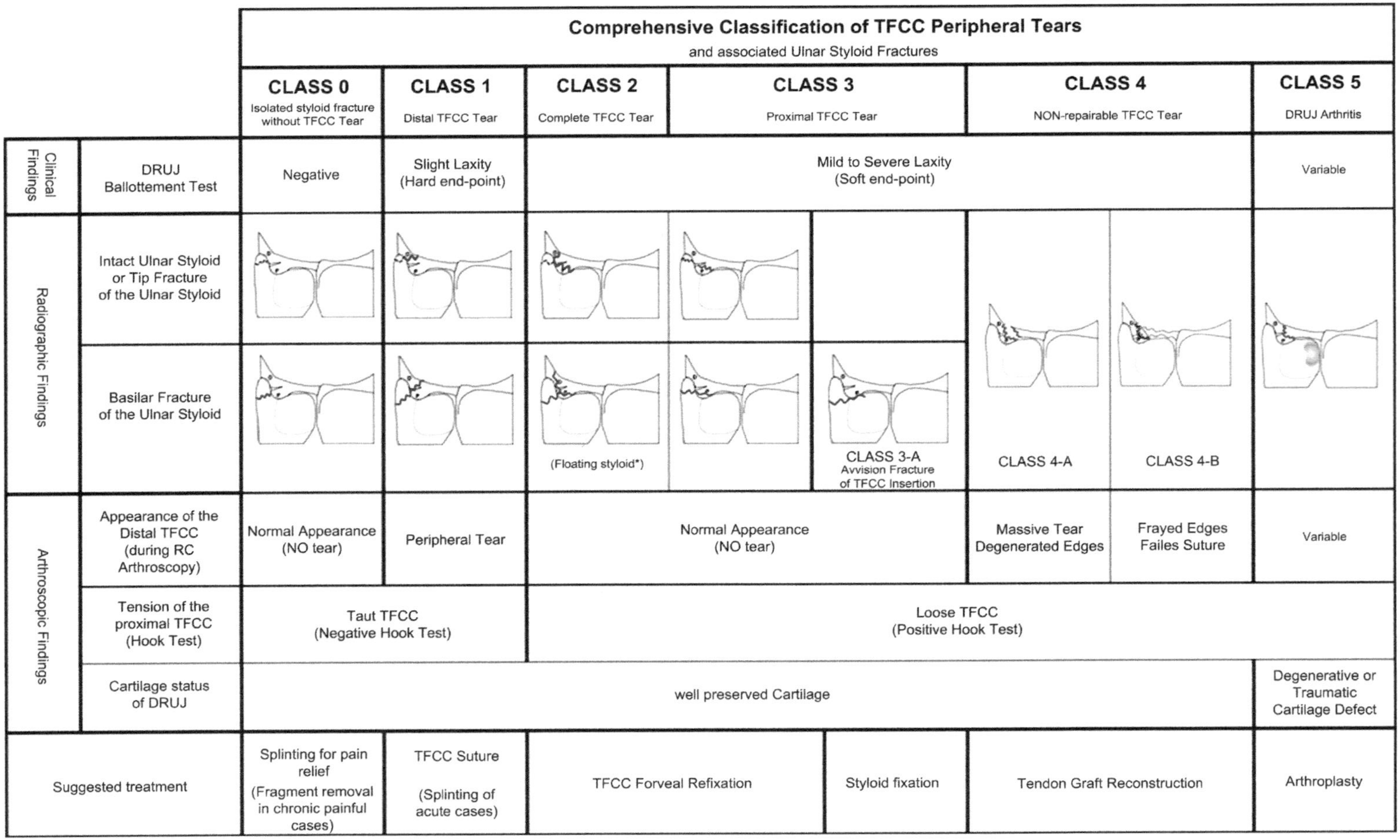

Comprehensive Classification of TFCC Peripheral Tears
and associated Ulnar Styloid Fractures

	CLASS 0 — Isolated styloid fracture without TFCC Tear	CLASS 1 — Distal TFCC Tear	CLASS 2 — Complete TFCC Tear	CLASS 3 — Proximal TFCC Tear	CLASS 4 — NON-repairable TFCC Tear		CLASS 5 — DRUJ Arthritis
Clinical Findings — DRUJ Ballottement Test	Negative	Slight Laxity (Hard end-point)	Mild to Severe Laxity (Soft end-point)				Variable
Radiographic Findings — Intact Ulnar Styloid or Tip Fracture of the Ulnar Styloid					CLASS 4-A	CLASS 4-B	
Radiographic Findings — Basilar Fracture of the Ulnar Styloid			(Floating styloid*)	CLASS 3-A Avulsion Fracture of TFCC Insertion			
Arthroscopic Findings — Appearance of the Distal TFCC (during RC Arthroscopy)	Normal Appearance (NO tear)	Peripheral Tear	Normal Appearance (NO tear)		Massive Tear Degenerated Edges	Frayed Edges Failes Suture	Variable
Arthroscopic Findings — Tension of the proximal TFCC (Hook Test)	Taut TFCC (Negative Hook Test)		Loose TFCC (Positive Hook Test)				
Arthroscopic Findings — Cartilage status of DRUJ	well preserved Cartilage						Degenerative or Traumatic Cartilage Defect
Suggested treatment	Splinting for pain relief (Fragment removal in chronic painful cases)	TFCC Suture (Splinting of acute cases)	TFCC Forveal Refixation	Styloid fixation	Tendon Graft Reconstruction		Arthroplasty

Fig. 11. Comprehensive classification of TFCC peripheral tears and associated ulnar styloid fracture. The classification system considers clinical, radiographic and arthroscopic findings. Clinical assessment of DRUJ instability is performed by the ballottement test. Radiographic findings are divided into two basic conditions according to the evidence of an intact ulnar styloid/tip fracture, or a basilar fracture of the ulnar styloid. Arthroscopy evaluates the TFCC by radiocarpal inspection and the hook test. DRU arthroscopy evaluates the cartilage of the sigmoid notch and ulnar head. Treatment is suggested according to the different Classes. See text.

arthroscopic suture to the ulnar wrist capsule or ECU tendon sheath.[10,38–40]

Class 2: Complete Peripheral TFCC Tear

A peripheral tear of the TFCC involves a laceration of both the distal and proximal component. The ballottement test demonstrates DRUJ laxity with a soft end point. Radiocarpal arthroscopy shows the distal peripheral tear, and the hook test is positive for a proximal TFCC disruption. The DRUJ cartilage is unaffected. The ulnar styloid may be intact, or fractured at the tip or mid-portion. Often the large ulnar styloid fragment may retain only a few ligamentous fibers. This particular condition is called a "floating styloid." In Class 2 lesions, the TFCC should be repaired to the fovea.[3,30] However, the floating styloid (the large styloid fragment with few ligamentous attachments) may require excision.

Class 3: Proximal Peripheral TFCC Tear

A Peripheral tear of the TFCC involves isolated laceration of a proximal component. The ballottement test demonstrates DRUJ laxity with a soft end point. The diagnosis of a Class 3 TFCC peripheral tear is often challenging because radiocarpal arthroscopy shows a normal, uninterrupted TFCC. However, the hook test is positive, suggesting a proximal TFCC disruption. DRU arthroscopy may be performed to confirm a foveal avulsion of the TFCC and the good quality of the cartilage. The ulnar styloid may be intact, or fractured at various levels. When the ulnar styloid is intact, when the fractured styloid is too small for internal fixation, or there is poor bone quality, TFCC foveal reattachment is recommended by transosseous sutures or a suture anchor.[3,7,9,26] The smaller or comminuted ulnar styloid is left in situ and rarely removed, though it may develop the radiographic appearance of a nonunion. When DRUJ instability is restored, the unrepaired or repaired ulnar styloid is seldom the cause of pain and it can be removed if it becomes symptomatic. However, a basilar fracture of the ulnar styloid that may occur following an avulsion injury from the proximal insertion of the TFCC can maintain its ligamentous attachments (Class 3-A). The persistence of a firm connection to the TFCC differentiates it from the floating styloid (Class 2) and provides the rationale for fixation with a small cannulated screw, K-wires, and/or tension band.

Class 4: Nonrepairable Peripheral TFCC Tear

A TFCC tear can be irreparable due to a sizable defect (Class 4-A) or poor healing potential (Class 4-B). The DRUJ is unstable. During radiocarpal arthroscopy, the TFCC may show a significant defect (Class 4-A), which may be due primarily to an extensive laceration following a high-energy injury or may result from the debridement that is required to refresh the degenerated or retracted TFCC tear's edges. Likewise, the TFCC tear may demonstrate frayed edges or elongated ligamentous remnants with reduced healing capacity (Class 4-B), due to ligamentous pathology or osseous dysmorphism or to the failure of a previous repair. Because cartilage erosion is likely to occur in long-standing conditions such as this, an accurate assessment of the quality of the DRUJ cartilage is mandatory. A nonrepairable TFCC tear requires reconstruction with a tendon graft, regardless of the presence of any ulnar styloid fracture.[10,29]

Class 5: DRUJ Arthritis Following Peripheral TFCC Tear

When DRU arthroscopy shows a significant degenerative or traumatic cartilage defect, the TFCC tear should not be repaired regardless of the variable clinical and arthroscopic findings. However, a resection arthroplasty or prosthetic replacement is recommended.[31–36]

REFERENCES

1. Palmer AK. Triangular fibrocartilage complex lesions: a classification. J Hand Surg Am 1989;14:594–606.
2. Nakamura T, Yabe Y, Horiuchi Y. Functional anatomy of the triangular fibrocartilage complex. J Hand Surg Br 1996;21:581–6.
3. Kleinman WB. Stability of the distal radioulnar joint: biomechanics, pathophysiology, physical diagnosis and restoration of function. What we have learned in 25 years. J Hand Surg Am 2007;32:1087–106.
4. Moritomo H, Murase T, Arimitsu S, et al. Change in the length of the ulnocarpal ligaments during radiocarpal motion: possible impact on triangular fibrocartilage complex foveal tears. J Hand Surg Am 2008;33:1278–86.
5. Estrella EP, Hung LK, Ho PC, et al. Arthroscopic repair of triangular fibrocartilage complex tears. Arthroscopy 2007;23:729–37.
6. Anderson ML, Larson AN, Moran SL, et al. Clinical comparison of arthroscopic versus open repair of triangular fibrocartilage complex tears. J Hand Surg Am 2008;33:675–82.
7. Chou KH, Sarris IK, Sotereanos DG. Suture anchor repair of ulnar-sided triangular fibrocartilage complex tears. J Hand Surg Br 2003;28:546–50.
8. Hermansdorfer JD, Kleinman WB. Management of chronic peripheral tears of the triangular fibrocartilage complex. J Hand Surg Am 1991;16:340–6.
9. Nakamura T, Nakao Y, Ikegami H, et al. Open repair of the ulnar disruption of the triangular fibrocartilage

complex with double three-dimensional mattress suturing technique. Tech Hand Up Extrem Surg 2004;8(2):116–23.

10. Atzei A. New trends in arthroscopic management of type 1-B TFCC injuries with DRUJ instability. J Hand Surg Eur Vol 2009;34(5):582–91.

11. Atzei A, Luchetti R. Clinical approach to the painful wrist. LLC. In: Geissler WB, editor. Wrist arthroscopy. New York: Springer-Verlag; 2005. p. 185–95.

12. Tay SC, Tomita K, Berger RA. The "ulnar fovea sign" for defining ulnar wrist pain: an analysis of sensitivity and specificity. J Hand Surg Am 2007;32(4):438–44.

13. Moriya T, Aoki M, Iba K, et al. Effect of triangular ligament tears on distal radioulnar joint instability and evaluation of three clinical tests: a biomechanical study. J Hand Surg Eur Vol 2009;34:219–23.

14. Lindau T, Adlercreutz C, Aspenberg P. Peripheral tears of the triangular fibrocartilage complex cause distal radioulnar joint instability after distal radial fractures. J Hand Surg Am 2000;25:464–8.

15. May MM, Lawton JN, Blazar PE. Ulnar styloid fractures associated with distal radius fractures: incidence and implications for distal radioulnar joint instability. J Hand Surg Am 2002;27:965–71.

16. Souer JS, Ring D, Matschke S, et al. Effect of an unrepaired fracture of the ulnar styloid base on outcome after plate-and-screw fixation of a distal radial fracture. J Bone Joint Surg Am 2009;91:830–8.

17. Hauck MR. Ulnar styloid fractures: a review. Curr Opin Orthop 2005;16:227–30.

18. Lindau T, Arner M, Hagberg L. Chondral and ligamentous wrist lesions in young adults with distal radius fractures. A descriptive, arthroscopic study in 50 patients. J Hand Surg Br 1997;22:638–43.

19. Lindau T. Treatment of injuries to the ulnar side of the wrist occurring with distal radial fractures. Hand Clin 2005;21:417–25.

20. Richards RS, Bennett JD, Roth JH, et al. Arthroscopic diagnosis of intraarticular soft tissue injuries associated with distal radial fractures. J Hand Surg Am 1997;22:772–6.

21. Pechlaner S, Kathrein A, Gabl M, et al. Distal radius fractures and concomitant injuries: experimental studies concerning pathomechanisms. J Hand Surg Eur Vol 2003;28:609–16.

22. Rettig ME, Raskin KB. Galeazzi fracture dislocation: a new treatment-oriented classification. J Hand Surg Am 2001;26:228–35.

23. Zanetti M, Bram J, Hodler J. Triangular fibrocartilage and intercarpal ligaments of the wrist: does MR arthrography improve standard MRI? J Magn Reson Imaging 1997;7(3):590–4.

24. Fulcher S, Poehling G. The role of operative arthroscopy for the diagnosis and treatment of lesions about the distal ulna. Hand Clin 1998;14:285–96.

25. Pederzini L, Luchetti R, Soragni O, et al. Evaluation of the triangular fibrocartilage complex tears by arthroscopy, arthrography, and magnetic resonance imaging. Arthroscopy 1992;8:191–7.

26. Atzei A, Luchetti R, Garcia-Elias M. Lesioni capsulo-legamentose della radio-ulnare distale e fibrocartilagine triangolare. In: Landi A, Catalano F, Luchetti R, editors. Trattato di Chirurgia della Mano. Roma (Italy): Verduci Editore Roma; 2006. p. 159–87 [in Italian].

27. Ruch DS, Yang CC, Smith BP. Results of acute arthroscopically repaired triangular fibrocartilage complex injuries associated with intra-articular distal radius fractures. Arthroscopy 2003;19:511–5.

28. Slutsky DJ. Clinical applications of volar portals in wrist arthroscopy. Tech Hand Up Extrem Surg 2004;8(4):229–38.

29. Adams BD. Anatomic reconstruction of the distal radioulnar ligaments for DRUJ instability. Tech Hand Up Extrem Surg 2000;4:154–60.

30. Atzei A, Rizzo A, Luchetti R, et al. Arthroscopic foveal repair of triangular fibrocartilage complex peripheral lesion with distal radioulnar joint instability. Tech Hand Up Extrem Surg 2008;12(4):226–35.

31. Garcia-Elias M. Eclypse: partial ulnar head replacement for the isolated distal radio-ulnar joint arthrosis. Tech Hand Up Extrem Surg 2007;11(1):121–8.

32. Laurentin-Perez LA, Goodwin AN, Babb BA, et al. A study of functional outcomes following implantation of a total distal radioulnar joint prosthesis. J Hand Surg Eur Vol 2008;33:18–28.

33. Sauvé L, Kapandji M. Nouvelle technique de traitement chirurgical des luxations recidivantes isolées de l'extrémité inferieure du cubitus. J Chir 1936;47:589–94 [in French].

34. Luchetti R, Khanchandani P, Da Rin F, et al. Arthroscopically assisted Sauvé-Kapandji procedure: an advanced technique for distal radioulnar joint arthritis. Tech Hand Up Extrem Surg 2008;12(4):216–20.

35. Luchetti R, Cozzolino R, Da Rin F, et al. Arthroscopic assisted Sauvé-Kapandji procedure. In: Herzberg G, editor. Avant-bras post-traumatique. Arthroscopie—arthroplasties. Montpellier (France): Sauramps Medical; 2009. p. 297–306.

36. Lluch A, Garcia-Elias M. The Sauvé-Kapandji procedure. In: Slutsky D, editor. Principles and practice of wrist surgery. Philadelphia: Saunders Elsevier; 2010. p. 335–44.

37. Giachino AA, McIntyre AI, Gui KJ, et al. Ulnar styloid triquetral impaction. Hand Surg 2007;12(2):123–34.

38. Pederzini LA, Tosi M, Prandini M, et al. All-class suture technique for Palmer class 1B triangular fibrocartilage repair. Riv Chir Mano 2006;43:1–3.

39. Poehling GP, Chabon SJ, Siegel DB. Diagnostic and operative arthroscopy. In: Gelberman RH, editor. The wrist: master techniques in orthopedic surgery. New York: Raven Press; 1994. p. 21–5.

40. Whipple TL, Geissler WB. Arthroscopic management of wrist triangular fibrocartilage complex injuries in the athlete. Orthopedics 1993;16:1061–7.

Arthroscopic Knotless Peripheral Ulnar-Sided TFCC Repair

William B. Geissler, MD

KEYWORDS

- Triangular fibrocartilage complex • Arthroscopy
- Knotless suture • Peripheral TFCC

Arthroscopy has continued to revolutionize the practice of orthopedic surgery, with the capability to visualize and treat intra-articular pathology. Arthroscopic surgery has continued to progress from its early stages involving the shoulder and knee to the smaller joints such as the wrist with the development of smaller instrumentation, arthroscopes, and new techniques. The wrist itself is a complex joint of 8 carpal bones with multiple articular surfaces combined with intrinsic and extrinsic ligaments, including the triangular fibro-cartilage complex (TFCC), all within a 5-cm interval. This perplexing joint continues to challenge physicians with its array of potential diagnoses and management. Wrist arthroscopy provides direct visualization of the cartilage surfaces, synovial tissue, and ligaments under bright light and magnified conditions. It has become a valuable adjunct in the management of disorders of the TFCC.

This article reviews the indications for wrist arthroscopy in the management of peripheral ulnar-sided tears of the articular disk involving the TFCC. Several techniques have been developed for repair of ulnar-sided tears of the articular disk,[1–4] which include both outside-in and inside-out techniques. These techniques primarily involve repair of the superficial layer of the articular disk. The techniques have been proved to be successful, but usually involve a small incision, and the suture knots can irritate the soft tissues during the repair. Recently, an all-arthroscopic knotless technique has been described for repair of peripheral ulnar-sided tears of the TFCC. The advantage of this technique is that it is entirely arthroscopic,

uses a suture anchor that does not require any knots to potentially irritate the soft tissues, allows for repair of both the superficial and deep layers off the articular disk, and the disk is repaired directly back down to bone. This article describes in detail this all-arthroscopic knotless technique.

The TFCC is a complex soft tissue structure that stabilizes the ulnar side of the wrist. It acts as an extension to the articular surface of the radius to support the proximal carpal row and also functions to stabilize the distal radioulnar joint. Classically, as described by Palmar, it has 4 components[5]: the fibrocartilage articular disk, the volar and dorsal radioulnar ligament, the meniscus homolog, and the floor of the tendon sheath of the extensor carpi ulnaris tendon. The central disk is wedge shaped in the coronal section, and sits radially by emerging with the hyaline cartilage of the sigmoid notch and the lunate facet of the distal radius.[6] The disk is relatively thinner on its radial attachment and thicker along its ulnar attachment.[7] Ulnarly, the articular disk has two bundles. One bundle is directed toward the ulnar styloid and the other to the fovea of the ulnar head. The proximal limbs of the volar and dorsal radioulnar ligaments conjoin and insert just medial to the ulnar styloid into the fovea. The deep layer has been commonly referred to as the ligamentum subcruentum. The superficial portions of the volar and dorsal radioulnar ligaments insert directly into the base of the ulnar styloid. The superficial and deep layers function independent of each other. The exact function of the superficial and deep components of the volar and dorsal radioulnar ligaments is controversial.

Division of Hand and Upper Extremity Surgery, Department of Orthopaedic Surgery and Rehabilitation, University of Mississippi Health Care, 2500 North State Street, Jackson, MS 39216, USA
E-mail address: 3doghill@msn.com

Hand Clin 27 (2011) 273–279
doi:10.1016/j.hcl.2011.05.008
0749-0712/11/$ – see front matter © 2011 Elsevier Inc. All rights reserved.

hand.theclinics.com

Dorsally the TFCC has attachments to the floor of the sheath of the extensor carpi ulnaris tendon, frequently an area of peripheral detachment of the articular disk. The floor of the sheath of the extensor carpi ulnaris is quite thick with stout, fibrous tissue. This stout tissue allows for firm fixation of the articular disk back to the floor of the sheath of the extensor carpi ulnaris.

The last component of the TFCC is described is the meniscus homolog, which is a controversial structure as to its function and existence. The meniscus homolog is a layer of fibrous connective tissue with variable thickness. This thickened layer of the meniscus homolog lies just dorsal to the prestyloid recess. It is important to understand that the prestyloid recess is a normal fovea and should not be mistaken for a peripheral tear of the articular disk. The prestyloid recess is the site for the 6-U portal, which is frequently used for inflow.

Though not initially described as contributing to the TFCC, the ulnocarpal ligaments are important stabilizers of the ulnar and palmar carpus. These ligaments are composed of the ulnolunate and ulnotriquetral ligaments, which insert independently on the lunate and triquetrum with additional insertion into the lunotriquetral osseous ligament. These ligaments originate from the palmar margin of the TFCC.

Thiru and colleagues[8] evaluated the arterial blood supply to the TFCC. Using latex injections, they determined there were 3 main arterial supplies to the complex itself. The ulnar artery supplies most of the blood to the TFCC, supporting the ulnar portion to dorsal and palmar radiocarpal branches. Thiru and colleagues noted that latex dye filled in the peripheral 15% to 20% of the articular disk. Bednar and colleagues,[9] in a similar study, found penetration of vessels into the peripheral 10% to 40% of the articular disk with an India-ink injection technique. These studies confirm an intact blood supply to the periphery of the articular disk and that, theoretically, peripheral tears to the articular disk have the ability to heal following repair.

DIAGNOSIS

Tears of the TFCC are common wrist injuries.[10] The most common mechanism occurs from a fall on the outstretched hand. Injuries to the TFCC usually occur with extension and pronation of an axially loaded carpus. Peripheral tears of the articular disk are common athletic injuries in sports that require rapid twisting and loading of the ulnar side of the wrist. It is common to see ulnar-sided wrist pain in golfers and athletes who play racquet sports. Peripheral ulnar-sided tears are also commonly seen in the workplace. Patients often describe a twisting or torquing of the forearm that may occur, for example, with the use of a power drill that suddenly binds, resulting in a twisting injury to the wrist.

Patients with ulnar-sided peripheral tears of the articular disk report they are point tender right at the prestyloid recess. This pain is increased with supination and pronation of the wrist. The pain may be further aggravated by anterior and posterior passive translation of the ulna in relation to the radius with the wrist in pronation and supination. Dorsal subluxation of the ulnar head in relation to the radius may be seen when a large peripheral tear is present. It is important to compare the opposite wrist when both wrists are in pronation and flexion.

DIAGNOSTIC MODALITIES

Patients who present with acute or chronic ulnar-sided wrist pain should be evaluated with standard anterior/posterior, lateral, and oblique radiographs of the wrist. It is important to take the anteroposterior view with the wrist in neutral position to evaluate for ulnar variance. The distal radioulnar joint should be evaluated for signs of ulnar impingement, which may be differentiated from pain arising from the TFCC. Radiographic signs of ulnar impaction, including cystic changes of the ulnar side of the lunate and of the ulnar head, should be looked for in patients who have an ulnar-positive wrist. In addition, signs of an acute fracture or nonunion of the ulnar styloid should be assessed on plain radiographs.

Triple-injection arthrography has traditionally been used in diagnosing tears of the TFCC.[11] Ulnar-sided peripheral tears of the articular disk, however, may be missed by arthrography, particularly in the chronic setting. This oversight is attributable to chronic synovitis that develops over the tear, which may block the flow of the dye between the radiocarpal and distal radioulnar joints.

More recently, magnetic resonance imaging (MRI) has been used to evaluate patients with a potential tear of the TFCC.[12,13] Pederzini and colleagues[14] compared arthrography, MRI, and arthroscopy in 11 patients with tears of the TFCC. Using arthroscopy as a gold standard, the investigators reported 100% specificity and 82% sensitivity by MRI evaluation.

Arthroscopy has a clear advantage in the evaluation of the articular disk under bright light and magnified conditions.[15] The tension of the articular disk can be palpated with a probe. A loss of tension may be detected in patients who have a peripheral tear when the articular disk is palpated with a probe. Frequently, reactive syno-vitis will have formed over the peripheral ulnar-sided tear; this needs to be debrided to clearly visualize the injury. A peripheral tear can be missed if any obscuring synovitis is not debrided. Arthroscopy not only has the advantage of being the most accurate modality in making the diag-nosis of peripheral tears of the articular disk, but may be used as an adjunct in its management as well.

In 1989 Palmar[5] proposed a classification system for tears of the TFCC, which divides in-juries into two basic categories: traumatic (Class I) and degenerative (Class II). Class I injuries are acute traumatic tears, which comprise the subject of this article. These tears are divided into 4 types based on the zone of injury. Type IA lesions involve a tear in the central avascular portion of the artic-ular disk and are therefore not suitable for suture repair. Type IB injuries (ulnar avulsion) occur when the ulnar side of the articular disk is avulsed from its insertion. These injuries may or may not be associated with a fracture of the ulnar styloid. These tears occur where there is a documented blood supply, and are very amenable to arthro-scopic repair. Type IC injuries involve a rupture of the volar attachment of the TFCC involving the ulnocarpal ligaments. Type ID (radial avulsion) occurs when the radial attachment of the articular disk as well as the radioulnar ligaments separate from the radius with or without a fracture of the radial sigmoid notch.

MANAGEMENT
Indications

Patients who present with ulnar-sided wrist pain with normal radiographs and with tenderness over the periphery of the TFCC are initially immobilized. Small ulnar peripheral tears of the articular disk potentially may heal with immobilization, due to its vigorous blood supply. Further diagnostic modalities are instituted after 2 or 3 months of immobilization if the patient continues to be symp-tomatic. Persistent ulnar-sided wrist pain not relieved by conservative management for at least 3 months is an indication for surgical intervention. Additional indications include symptomatic distal radioulnar joint instability that is not relieved by immobilization. Individuals contraindicated for surgical management include patients who are minimally symptomatic despite the radiographic findings, patients with low physical demands who are not healthy enough for surgery, and patients who have degenerative changes of either the radio-carpal or distal radioulnar joint. These patients may be better managed by other modalities.

Arthroscopic Knotless Peripheral TFCC Repair

The wrist is suspended in 10 lb (4.5 kg) of traction in a traction tower. The volar arm and forearm are well padded with towels so that no portion of the skin comes in contact directly with the tower itself. This action is taken is to prevent any potential burns from the heat of the tower that has just been sterilized. Inflow is provided with a needle in either the 6-U portal or 1–2 portal. Frequently, the 1–2 portal is used for inflow so that the inflow cannula will be out of the way during the arthro-scopic peripheral TFCC repair. The 3–4 portal is identified initially with an 18-gauge needle, then the skin only is incised with the tip of a number 11 blade. Blunt dissection is continued with a hemostat to the level of the capsule, and the arthroscope with a blunt trocar is then introduced into the 3–4 portal. An 18-gauge needle is used to identify the exact location of the 6-R portal just distal to the articular disk. This action prevents accidental injury to the articular disk or damage to the articular cartilage of the lunate or triquetrum. The 6-R portal is made once the ideal portal loca-tion is determined. The integrity of the triangular fi-brocartilage (TFC) is then inspected. It is important to palpate the articular disk and evaluate the loss of tension when a peripheral tear is present. Syno-vitis about the periphery of the ulnar-sided tear is debrided to fully visualize the extent of the periph-eral ulnar-sided tear.

An accessory 6-R portal is made approximately 1.5 cm distally in line with the traditional 6-R portal. This portal is located by using an 18-gauge needle inserted through the skin and aimed at the fovea of the ulnar head (Fig. 1). The ulnar head should be palpated with the needle. Once the ideal location of the accessory 6-R portal has been identified, the portal is established. It is helpful to have the wrist flexed about 20° to 30° for easier access to the base of the ulna through the accessory 6-R portal. The skin only is incised when making the accessory 6-R portal in order to protect the dorsal sensory branch of the ulnar nerve. Blunt dissection is performed with a hemostat to the capsule, which is then opened.

A suture lasso is inserted through the accessory 6-R portal into the radiocarpal space (Fig. 2). The curve of the suture lasso is placed underneath the torn edge of the TFC and then used to pierce through the articular disk in a proximal to distal direction. It is helpful to gently twist the lasso between the thumb and index finger to ease its penetration through the tough tissue of the artic-ular disk (Fig. 3). Both the superficial and deep layers of the articular disk are pierced through with the suture lasso. A wire suture passer is

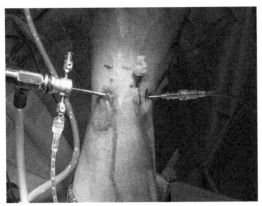

Fig. 1. Outside view demonstrating the arthroscope in the 3–4 portal. Inflow is brought in through the needle through the 6-U, and the 6-R portal has been made. The ideal location for the accessory 6-R portal is made by inserting a needle approximately 1.5 cm distal to the 6-R portal and palpating the fovea of the ulna.

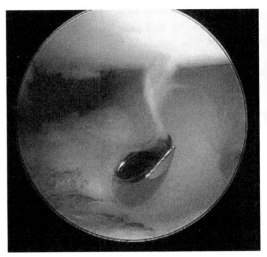

Fig. 3. The suture lasso pierces through both the superficial and deep layers of the articular disk, as seen with the arthroscope in the 3–4 portal.

then inserted through the suture lasso and removed through the 6-R portal with a grasper (**Fig. 4**). A 2.0 fiber wire suture (Arthrex, Naples, FL, USA) is placed through the wire suture retriever and pulled distally through the suture lasso and outward (**Fig. 5**). The suture lasso is then backed out of the articular disk and reinserted either anterior or posterior to the original perforation so that a horizontal mattress-type suture is placed. A loop of suture is formed that protrudes through the articular disk into the radiocarpal space as the suture lasso pierces the articular disk for a second time (**Fig. 6**). This loop of suture is then retrieved through the 6-R portal with a suture grasper so that both limbs are exiting the 6-R portal (**Fig. 7**).

A cannula is then inserted through the accessory 6-R portal. The suture-wire retriever is inserted through the cannula and passed out through the 6-R portal with a grasper. The two suture limbs are then placed into the loop of the suture-wire retriever and pulled through the cannula exiting the accessory 6-R portal (**Fig. 8**). Both suture limbs are now exiting the cannula through the accessory 6-R portal. The cannula is then pressed down firmly onto the head of the ulna and the sutures are pulled through the slot of the cannula, so as not to interfere with drilling of the ulnar head.

At this point the surgeon has two options. A cannulated trocar may be inserted through the cannula and a Kirschner wire inserted into the

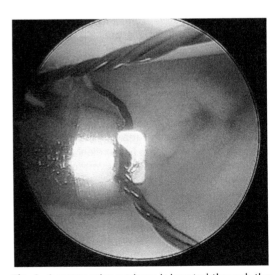

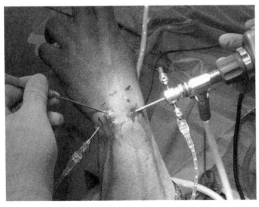

Fig. 2. Outside view demonstrating insertion of the suture lasso through the accessory 6-R portal.

Fig. 4. A suture-wire retriever is inserted through the suture lasso and grabbed out with a suture grasper through the 6-R portal.

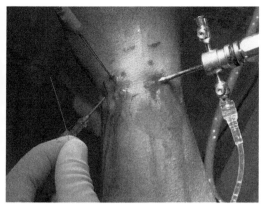

Fig. 5. Outside view demonstrating the passage of the wire retriever outward through the 6-R portal. A 2.0 fiber wire (Arthrex, Naples, FL, USA) is inserted through the loop of the suture lasso.

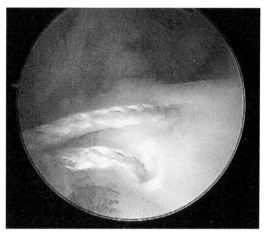

Fig. 7. With a suture grasper, this loop of suture is pulled out through the 6-R portal so both limbs of the suture are exiting this portal.

ulnar head. The position of the Kirschner guide wire may then be checked under fluoroscopy to ensure the insertion point of the anchor will be at the fovea of the ulna. A cannulated drill is inserted over the guide wire and a drill hole is made in the base of the ulna after the ideal location of the guide wire has been confirmed under fluoroscopy. Alternatively, if the surgeon feels comfortable that the cannula is in the ideal foveal location by palpation, the fovea may be drilled. It is important to keep the cannula in the exact same location once the ulna has been drilled. The suture limbs are then inserted through a mini push lock anchor (Arthrex) and the anchor is advanced down the cannula into the drill hole (Fig. 9). The sutures are tensioned and the push-lock anchor is advanced into the ulnar head (Figs. 10 and 11). The tendency is to

slide off the ulna volarly and miss the drill hole. Once the anchor has been inserted, tension is placed on the handle and the sutures to make sure the anchor cannot be pulled out of the bone. If there is resistance, the anchors have been correctly inserted into the bone. If the anchor misses the bone, the anchor will easily pull out of the soft tissues with tension on the handle. The sutures are then cut with a small upbiter inserted through the 6-R portal and the inserter is removed from the anchor (Fig. 12). This action completes the repair of the articular disk back down to bone with an all-arthroscopic knotless technique (Fig. 13).

The wrist is then immobilized in slight supination in an above-elbow splint for 4 weeks. A removable wrist splint is then used for an additional 3 weeks. Digital range-of-motion exercises are started immediately. Range-of-motion and strengthening exercises of the forearm and wrist are initiated at

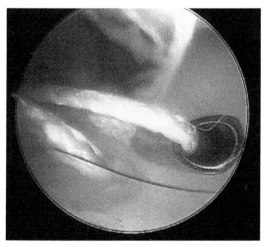

Fig. 6. The 2.0 fiber wire is pulled out through the proximal aspect of the suture lasso. The suture lasso is then used to reperforate through the articular disk and a loop of suture is formed.

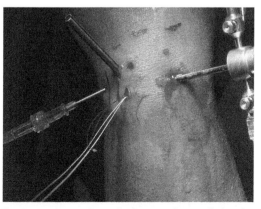

Fig. 8. A wire retriever is then used to pull the two suture limbs from the 6-R portal through the cannula, exiting out of the accessory 6-R portal.

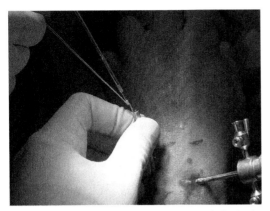

Fig. 9. The fovea of the ulna has been drilled. The cannula is held firmly against the head of the ulna. The two suture limbs are inserted through the mini knotless anchor (Arthrex) and the anchor is inserted through the cannula.

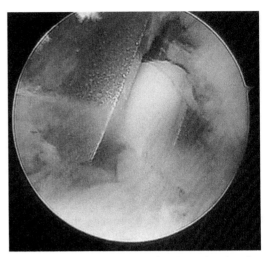

Fig. 11. Arthroscopic view showing the knotless anchor (Arthrex) being inserted intra-articularly into the base of the ulna.

7 weeks. Most patients are discharged at approximately 3 months postoperatively.

DISCUSSION

Trauma of the ulnar side of the wrist usually involves a spectrum of injury. A peripheral ulnar-sided tear of the articular disk may be the first stage of a complex multifactorial ligamentous injury. In addition to ulnar-sided wrist pain, patients may present with signs and symptoms of distal radioulnar joint instability in larger tears. Arthroscopic evaluation is an important adjunct in the management of these complex injuries, particularly when diagnostic studies are normal and the clinician strongly suspects a soft tissue injury to the TFCC. Current arthroscopic techniques for repair of peripheral ulnar-sided tears of the articular disk have been shown to have good results, as seen in the literature. Corso and

colleagues[16] reported the results of a multicenter study of patients who underwent the Whipple technique and did not have a foveal repair. The investigators noted 41 of 45 patients with good or excellent results using the Mayo modified wrist score. Fulcher and Poehling[15] reported results using the Tuohy technique, and noted a 70% satisfaction rate after 6 to 24 months in 17 patients. Estrella and colleagues[3] reviewed their results in 35 patients who were repaired using either the Whipple or Tuohy needle procedure. Using the Mayo modified wrist score they found that 74% of the patients had good or excellent results.

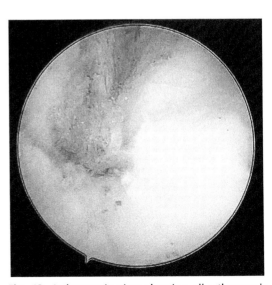

Fig. 12. Arthroscopic view showing all-arthroscopic knotless repair of the periphery of the articular disk back down to bone, restoring tension to the articular disk.

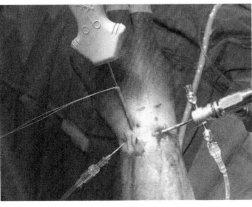

Fig. 10. The handle is used to insert the anchor into the previously drilled hole into the fovea of the ulna.

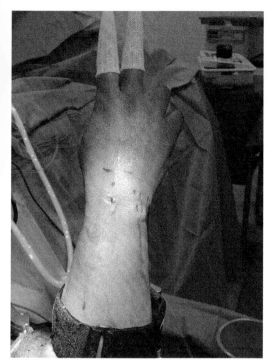

Fig. 13. Exterior view showing the 3 arthroscopic portals used for arthroscopic knotless peripheral repair of the articular disk.

While these current arthroscopic techniques for peripheral tears of the TFCC have been shown to be successful in the literature, patients may complain of pain around the suture knots. Patients may complain of pain with pronation and supination over the extensor carpi ulnaris tendon sheath after undergoing the Whipple technique. The dorsal sensory branch of the ulnar nerve is put at risk with the Tuohy needle technique.

The all-arthroscopic knotless technique has several advantages. This technique allows for repair of both the superficial and deep layers of the TFCC back down to bone. In patients who present with instability of the distal radioulnar joint, repair of the articular disk back down to bone may be desired. Repair of both layers of the articular disk back down to bone may provide greater stability. In addition, there is no irritation of the suture knots in comparison with previous techniques. The technique that is performed purely arthroscopically does not require an incision over the extensor carpi ulnaris tendon that could cause potential instability to the tendon sheath. Also, risk of injury to the dorsal sensory branch of the ulnar nerve is minimized as compared with other techniques.

Potential further refinements in wrist arthroscopy techniques such as those described in this article will further enhance the management of wrist injuries and improve patients' satisfaction and outcome.

REFERENCES

1. Trumble TE, Gilbert M, Vedder N. Isolated tears of the triangular fibrocartilage: management by early arthroscopic repair. J Hand Surg 1997;22:57–65.
2. de Araujo W, Poehling G, Kuzma G. New Tuohy needle technique for triangular fibrocartilage complex repair: preliminary studies. Arthroscopy 1996;12:699–703.
3. Estrella EP, Hung LK, Ho PC, et al. Arthroscopic repair of triangular fibrocartilage complex tears. Arthroscopy 2007;23(7):729–37.
4. Ruch DS, Papadonikolakis A. Arthroscopically assisted repair of peripheral triangular fibrocartilage complex tears: factors affecting outcome. Arthroscopy 2005;21(9):1126–30.
5. Palmar AK. Triangular fibrocartilage complex lesions: a classification. J Hand Surg 1989;14:594–606.
6. Chidgey LK, Dell PC, Bittar ES, et al. Histologic anatomy of the triangular fibrocartilage. J Hand Surg 1991;16:1084–100.
7. Adams B. Partial excision of the triangular fibrocartilage complex articular disk, a biomechanical study. J Hand Surg 1993;184:334–40.
8. Thiru RG, Ferlic DC, Clayton MI, et al. Arterial anatomy of the triangular fibrocartilage of the wrist and its surgical significance. J Hand Surg 1986;11:258–63.
9. Bednar MS, Arnoczky SP, Weiland AJ. The microvasculature of the triangular fibrocartilage complex: its clinical significance. J Hand Surg 1991;16:1101–5.
10. Cooney WP, Linscheid RL, Dobyns JH. Triangular fibrocartilage tears. J Hand Surg 1994;19:143–54.
11. Weiss A, Akelman E, Lambiase R. Comparison of the findings of triple-injection cinearthrography of the wrist with those of arthroscopy. J Bone Joint Surg Am 1996;78:348–56.
12. Golimbu C, Firooznia H, Melone CJ, et al. Tears of the triangular fibrocartilage of the wrist: MR imaging. Radiology 1989;173:731–3.
13. Skahen JI, Palmer A, Levinsohn E, et al. Magnetic resonance imaging of the triangular fibrocartilage complex. J Hand Surg 1990;15A:552–7.
14. Pederzini L, Luchetti R, Soragni O, et al. Evaluation of the triangular fibrocartilage complex by arthroscopy, arthrography, and magnetic resonance imaging. Arthroscopy 1992;8:191–7.
15. Fulcher S, Poehling G. The role of operative arthroscopy for the diagnosis and treatment of lesions about the distal ulna. Hand Clin 1998;14:285–96.
16. Corso S, Savoie F, Geissler W, et al. Arthroscopic repair of peripheral avulsions of the triangular fibrocartilage complex of the wrist: a multicenter study. Arthroscopy 1997;13:78–84.

Repair of Foveal Detachment of the Triangular Fibrocartilage Complex: Open and Arthroscopic Transosseous Techniques

Toshiyasu Nakamura, MD, PhD*, Kazuki Sato, MD, PhD,
Masato Okazaki, MD, Yoshiaki Toyama, MD, PhD,
Hiroyasu Ikegami, MD, PhD

KEYWORDS

- Triangular fibrocartilage complex • Foveal tear
- Arthroscopic repair • Open repair • DRUJ instability

ANATOMY OF THE TFCC

The triangular fibrocartilage complex (TFCC) consists of the triangular fibrocartilage (TFC; also termed the articular disc or disc proper),[1–3] meniscus homolog, the radioulnar ligament (RUL),[1,2,4,5] ulnolunate ligament, ulnotriquetral ligament, the extensor carpi ulnaris (ECU) subsheath,[6] and the ulnar joint capsule.[2,7,8] This complex allows smooth motion of the wrist and forearm, distributes load between the ulna and ulnar carpus, and stabilizes the ulnocarpal joint as well as the distal radioulnar joint (DRUJ). The TFCC is divided into 3 components three-dimensionally: The distal hammocklike structure includes the centrally located fibrocartilage disc, meniscus homolog, ulnolunate ligament, and ulnotriquetral ligament, which support and surrounds the ulnar carpus; the RUL, which is the proximal component of the TFCC that stabilizes the radius to the ulna directly,[5] and the functional ulnar collateral ligament, which consists of the sheath floor of the ECU and the thickened ulnar capsule.[2,7,8] The histology of the TFCC shows that the RUL originates from the wide area of the fovea and base of the ulnar styloid nearly vertically (**Fig. 1**), then curls radially and separates into palmar and dorsal portions that pass through the proximal portion of the TFCC,[2] eventually attaching to the radial edge of the sigmoid notch (see **Fig. 1**).[7,8]

During pronation-supination, the RUL is twisted at its origin at the fovea.[2,8] Centrally originating fibers from the fovea in both the dorsal and palmar portions of the RUL show a nearly isometric length pattern. However, the fibers originating from the eccentric area in the fovea and base of the ulnar styloid reveal changes in the length: the eccentric dorsal fibers are longer in pronation and shorter in supination; the eccentric

The authors have nothing to disclose.
Department of Orthopaedic Surgery, School of Medicine, Keio University, 35 Shinanomachi, Shinjuku-ku, Tokyo 160-8582, Japan
* Corresponding author.
E-mail address: tosiyasu@sc.itc.keio.ac.jp

Hand Clin 27 (2011) 281–290
doi:10.1016/j.hcl.2011.05.002

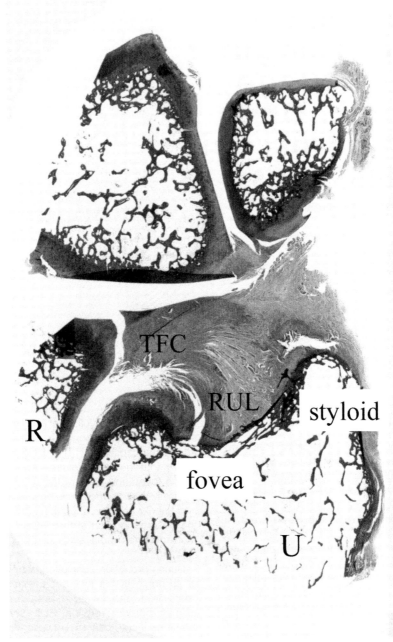

Fig. 1. Histologic section of the TFCC. Note that the radioulnar ligament (RUL) arises from wide area from fovea to the base of the ulnar styloid. Main attaching portion of the TFCC is the fovea. R, radius; U, ulna.

palmar fibers are longer in supination and shorter in pronation.[5]

PATHOLOGY OF THE FOVEAL DETACHMENT OF THE TFCC

Palmer[9] classified TFCC tears into traumatic (class 1) and degenerative (class 2) tears. Traumatic TFCC tear were also subclassified as central tears (1A), ulnar tears (1B), distal tears (1C), and radial tears (1D) based on the clinical patterns seen through radiocarpal (RC) arthroscopy.[9] Palmer 1B tears are peripheral ulnar tears of the TFCC that may be associated with an ulnar styloid fracture because the TFCC had been considered to attach only to the ulnar styloid. The TFCC is anchored to the DRUJ via the RUL, which attaches to the ulnar fovea and base of the ulnar styloid, hence a hyper-rotation force or dislocation force applied to the RUL from the ulnar head, such as in a fall, may disrupt the RUL not only from the ulnar styloid but also from the fovea. Because the fovea has a larger attaching area than the base of the ulnar styloid, avulsion at the fovea may indicate greater instability.[10] Once the TFCC is detached from the fovea, DRUJ instability must occur. A horizontal tear or proximal slit-type tear of the TFCC may also occur through the same mechanism of injury.

A foveal detachment of the TFCC is clearly evident in clinical practice. Atzei[11] recently subclassified the Palmer 1B tear into a distal component, a proximal component, or both (complete). An isolated foveal detachment is equivalent to a proximal component tear.

Recent anatomic and biomechanical findings have advanced our knowledge on repair methods for a foveal disruption of the TFCC.[5,7,8] The TFCC can be described as a hammock that surrounds and supports the carpus, with 2 tight anchors to the fovea. Once the anchors are disrupted, the hammock is unsteady. DRUJ stability can be achieved by reanchoring the RUL. The direction of the sutures must be parallel to direction of the vertical RUL fibers. Because of the isometricity,[5] the fibers must be attached at the center of the fovea. If the eccentric fibers are repaired, the sutures may tear, elongate, or cause a severe loss of forearm rotation.

TREATMENT OPTIONS FOR FOVEAL TEAR OF THE TFCC

In the positive ulnar variance wrist, the ulnar shortening procedure successfully reduces the pressure between the ulna and ulnar carpus.[12,13] Thus it is indicated in a degenerative tear of the TFCC in the presence of an ulnocarpal abutment syndrome.[9] The ulnar shortening may also stabilize the DRUJ because the TFCC is tightened by the pulling effect from the shortened ulna. However, it can no longer stabilize the DRUJ biomechanically in the presence of a complete avulsion of the TFCC at the fovea.[14] An ulnar shortening osteotomy is not indicated in an ulnar minus variance wrist because of the decrease of adaptation area of the DRUJ and increase of pressure between the DRUJ.[15]

During the last decade, arthroscopic[16–21] or open repair[22–25] techniques for ulnar disruptions of the TFCC have been reported. Avulsion of the TFCC from the fovea may induce DRUJ instability,[10] but the conventional arthroscopic capsular repair technique of the TFCC to the dorsal or ulnar joint capsule[17–19] most commonly used to repair this foveal disruption does not reconstitute the foveal

origin, where the RUL arises. There are 2 recent papers on arthroscopic assisted transosseous repair techniques of the TFCC. Atzei and colleagues[20] explored the foveal lesion arthroscopically and then used an open technique to reattach the foveal insertion using bone anchor. Iwasaki and Minami[21] used a 2.9-mm drill hole made from the proximal ulnar cortex to the fovea under fluoroscopic control with an arthroscopically assisted suture of the TFCC to the ulnar periosteum.[21]

In previous reports of open repair, the TFCC was considered a two-dimensional flat shape, and the TFCC was reattached by single pull-out technique[22,23] or suture anchor.[24,25] We have described a three-dimensional mattress suture technique, in which the sutures are placed in an anatomic orientation that is parallel to the RUL fiber direction, inserting on the isometric point at the center of the fovea.[26]

DIAGNOSIS OF THE FOVEAL TFCC TEAR

There are several physical testing maneuvers that can be used to detect a TFCC tear, including the ulnocarpal stress test, the fovea sign, and the DRUJ instability test. The ulnocarpal stress test is effective for assessment of a TFCC tear, but has a low specificity for a foveal tear. The fovea sign consists of tenderness to palpation along the ulnar capsule at the base of the ulnar styloid surrounded by the ECU and flexor carpi ulnaris tendons, and suggests an ulnocarpal split tear. It may also be present with a foveal detachment.[27] The most reliable physical test is the DRUJ instability test, in which the dorsopalmar stability between the ulna and radius is examined in the neutral, pronated, and supinated positions, respectively.[28] When the fovea is intact, there is a stable end point, whereas, with a complete foveal detachment, there is no end point, and there may be multidirectional instability of the DRUJ. The piano-key sign, which consists of dorsal instability of the ulnar head with the wrist in pronation, may also be positive.

Magnetic resonance imaging (MRI) can show a TFCC tear including a foveal detachment (Fig. 2). A gradient echo sequence T2*-weighted image and a fat-suppression T1-weighted image provide a high-delineation image of the TFCC structure.[29] A recent high-resolution technique is now available.[30] In the foveal detachment of the TFCC, the arthrogram shows pooling of the dye between the TFCC and ulnar fovea (Fig. 3).

DRUJ ARTHROSCOPY

RC arthroscopy can only show a loss of trampoline effect as well as a loss of the peripheral tension

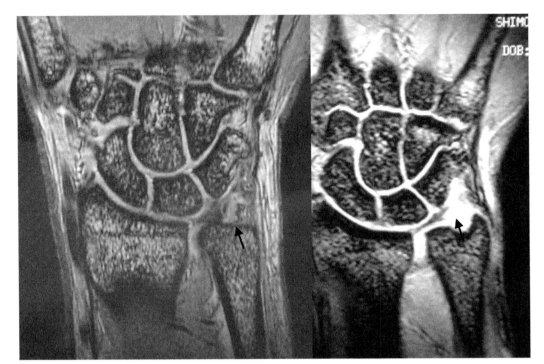

Fig. 2. Typical MRI of foveal detachment of the TFCC. Note high signal intensity area at the fovea with an absence of a low signal ligament structure (*arrows*).

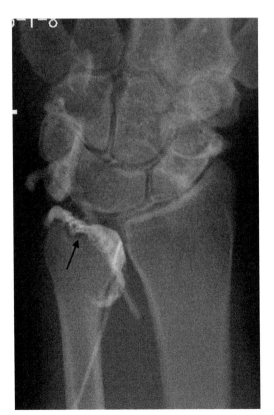

Fig. 3. Arthrogram of foveal avulsion. Dye passing from the DRUJ to the ulnar side of the ulnar styloid through the fovea indicates a complete foveal avulsion (*arrow*).

(positive hook test)[11] of the disc in patients with a foveal disruption, because the TFCC is no longer connected to the ulna. When the distal hammock-like structure of the TFCC surrounding the carpus is intact, the peripheral tension of the TFC is intact. In contrast, DRUJ arthroscopy can directly show a complete foveal rupture of the TFCC (**Fig. 4**). In a foveal detachment, the foveal region can easily be seen through DRUJ arthroscopy, because the DRUJ is loose. When the TFCC is well attached to the ulna with no DRUJ instability, the foveal area is difficult to visualize even with DRUJ arthroscopy. There are several findings that may be seen during DRUJ arthroscopy in the presence of a foveal detachment, including an absent RUL, which is sometimes replaced by scar tissue, attenuation of the RUL, or a partial tear either on the dorsal or palmar portion of the RUL.

ARTHROSCOPIC TRANSOSSEOUS REPAIR

We reserve the arthroscopic repair technique for a fresh (up to 6 months after the initial injury) complete or partial ulnar disruption of the TFCC at the fovea. The technique described is suited for wrists with an ulnar neutral or minus variance. In the wrists with a positive ulnar variance, shear stress between the ulnar head and the suture site of the TFCC may rupture the sutures.

The concept of this technique is based on the anatomic characteristics of the TFCC, in which

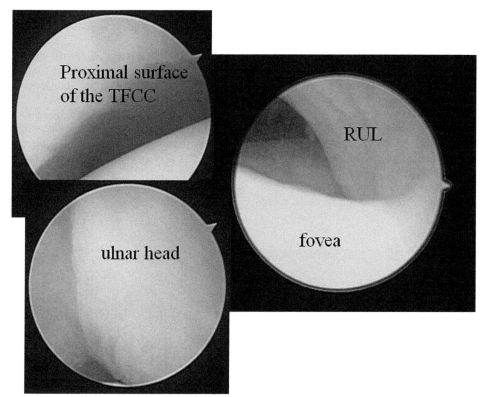

Fig. 4. DRUJ arthroscopy offers direct vision of the ulnar head, radial sigmoid notch, proximal surface of the TFCC, fovea, and RUL. This case shows an absence of the foveal ligament, which is replaced by scar tissue.

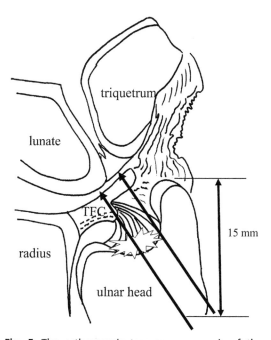

Fig. 5. The arthroscopic transosseous repair of the TFCC. The line between a point on the ulnar cortex of the ulnar shaft 15 mm proximal to the tip of the ulnar styloid and the ulnar half of the TFC passes through the fovea lesion. If the sutures are introduced into this area, theoretically the TFCC can be sutured to the fovea with outside-in pull-out technique.

a line drawn between a point on the ulnar cortex of the ulnar shaft 15 mm proximal to the tip of the ulnar styloid and the ulnar half of the TFC passes through the foveal insertion, which is the isometric point of forearm rotation (**Fig. 5**). First, the TFCC is observed via RC and DRUJ arthroscopy. RC arthroscopy sometimes shows an intact TFC (no tear) or just a radial-sided tear of the TFC. DRUJ arthroscopy shows variable disorders of the RUL at the fovea. After a foveal detachment of the TFCC is confirmed, the target device (**Fig. 6**; Nakashima Medical, Okayama, Japan) is inserted through the 4/5 or 6R portal and a 1-cm longitudinal incision is made on the ulnar side of the ulnar

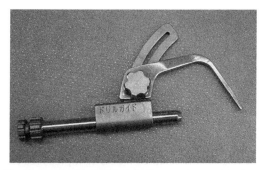

Fig. 6. Original targeting device.

cortex, just 15 mm proximal to the tip of the ulnar styloid, and the periosteum elevated. The small spike on the target device is set on the ulnar half of the TFC. Two separate small holes with 1.2-mm K-wires are made from the ulnar cortex of the ulna to the ulnar half of the TFC. DRUJ arthroscopy is helpful to confirm accurate placement of the drill holes at the fovea. A looped nylon 4-0 suture is passed through a 21-gauge needle that is passed through one tunnel from the outside, then is repeated through the other bone tunnel (**Fig. 7**). Both loop sutures are retrieved through the 4/5 or 6R portal using blunt mosquito forceps, then 2 nonabsorbable 3-0 polyester sutures (Ticron, Covidien, Mansfield, MA, USA) are threaded through the loop sutures and introduced into the RC joint. Proximal traction on the looped sutures then pulls the polyester sutures through the TFCC and out the ulnar cortex of the ulna advancing the TFCC to the fovea (see **Fig. 7**). The TFCC is tightly sutured to the ulnar fovea with this technique, which restabilizes the DRUJ.

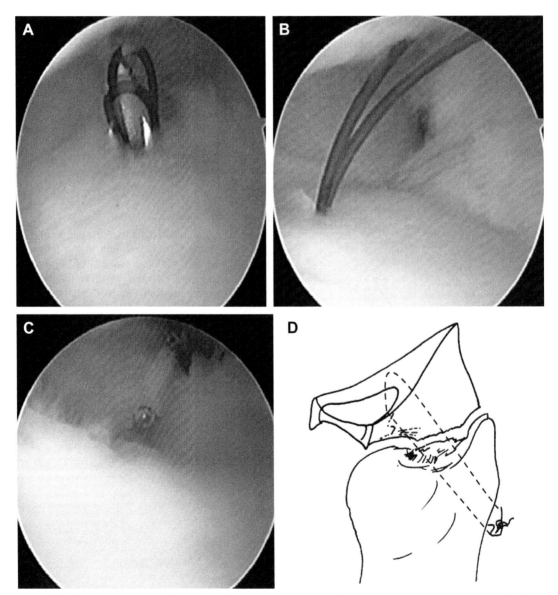

Fig. 7. (*A*) A 21-gauge needle with a loop nylon 4-0 suture is passed from the ulnar cortex to the ulnar half area of the TFC. (*B*) Two nonabsorbable 3-0 polyester sutures are introduced from the RC joint to the ulnar cortex of the ulna. (*C*) The detached TFCC is tightly repaired to the fovea. (*D*) Arthroscopic transosseous repair of the TFCC. Dashed line indicates the suture.

OPEN TRANSOSSEOUS REPAIR OF THE TFCC

An open repair is suitable for a fresh to subacute (up to 1 year after the initial injury) avulsion of the TFCC at the fovea, in which there is severe DRUJ instability. A positive ulnar variance is corrected to a neutral variance before repairing the TFCC by performing an ulnar shortening osteotomy.[26]

A dorsal C-shaped skin incision is used, extending from the 4/5 or 6R portal for RC arthroscopy and/or from the DRUJ portal for DRUJ arthroscopy with the forearm suspended by finger traps. After the C-flap is elevated, the superficial sensory branches of the ulnar nerve should be preserved. The sixth extensor compartment is opened and the ECU is retracted. After the radial ridge of the ECU subsheath is released, the dorsal DRUJ capsule is elevated from the ulnar head with a scalpel to expose the DRUJ. A small ring elevator is inserted into the DRUJ to dislocate the ulnar head (**Fig. 8**), which is easy if there is foveal disruption of the TFCC.[26]

A foveal tear of the TFCC and/or the RUL is clearly visible by making an additional 5-mm longitudinal incision at the origin of the RUL. The condition of the fibers of the RUL can be assessed by pulling the distal remnant with a pair of forceps to determine whether it can be sutured. The fovea of the ulna is debrided of scar tissue and 2 small holes are made with a 1.2-mm K-wire, as close to the center of the fovea as possible, which is an isometric point on the ulna during forearm rotation. Using the 21-gauge needles, two 3-0 nylon or polyester sutures are passed through the first bone hole from the ulnar fovea to the lateral cortex of the ulna. The disrupted RUL is sutured with double three-dimensional mattress and a locking suture technique (**Fig. 9**). The ECU is reduced to the sheath, which is then repaired. The dorsal DRUJ capsule is anatomically repaired with closure of the ECU sheath.

POSTOPERATIVE COURSE

Two weeks of long arm casting with the forearm in neutral rotation and 3 weeks of short arm casting are necessary. After removal of the cast at 5 weeks after surgery, active range of motion (ROM) exercise begin. Seven weeks after the operation, passive ROM exercises under the direction of an occupational therapist may be needed if there is a loss of pronation-supination. Usually, at 8 to 9 weeks after the operation, full pronation-supination range is achieved, and then isometric strengthening exercises begin with up to a 3-kg weight. The wrist must be held in the neutral position during the exercise. Three months after the operation, the weight can be increased to 5 kg. The patient may resume sports activities 6 months after the surgery.

PATIENT SERIES

We treated 24 wrists with an arthroscopic transosseous repair technique and 66 wrists with a TFCC tear with an open transosseous repair. In the arthroscopic repair group, there were 13 male and 11 female, with a mean age of 27 years. The injured side included 13 right and 11 left wrists. A period between the initial injury and an operation averaged 8 months (range 1 month to 4 years). The ulnar variance was +2 mm in 5 wrists, 0 mm in 17 wrists, and −1 mm in 2 wrists. The follow-up averaged 3.5 years (range 12 to 60 months). In the open repair group, there were 36 male and 28 female, with a mean age of 31 years. The injured side included 37 right wrists, 25 left wrists, and 2 bilateral. The period between the initial injury and the operation averaged 5 months (range 0 month to 25 years). Ulnar variance was positive in 13 wrists, neutral in 50 wrists, and minus in 3 wrists. The follow-up averaged 3 years (range 24 to 108 months). All cases in both groups were consistent with a foveal detachment at the

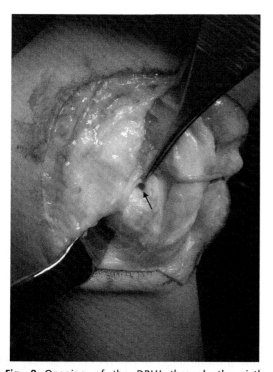

Fig. 8. Opening of the DRUJ through the sixth compartment. The ring retractor is inserted to dislocate the ulnar head. Arrow indicates an avulsion of the TFCC at the fovea.

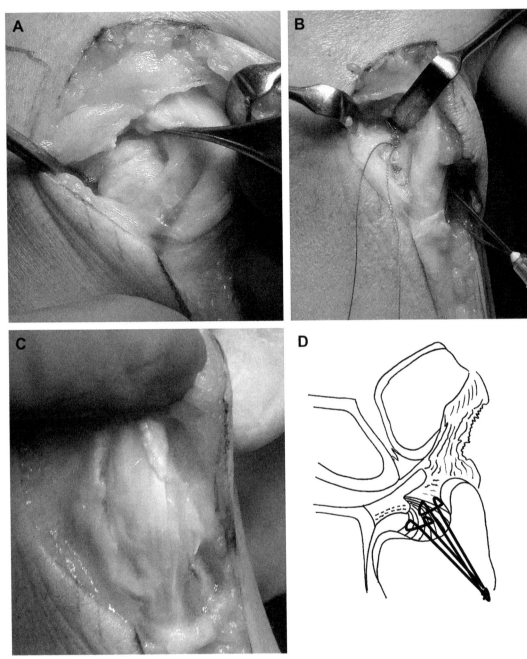

Fig. 9. (*A*) The condition of the RUL is checked with forceps. (*B*) Two nonabsorbable 3-0 polyester sutures are introduced from the fovea to the ulnar cortex of the ulna. (*C*) TFCC is tightly repaired to the fovea with open pull-out technique. (*D*) An open transosseous repair of the TFCC. Solid lines represent the sutures.

TFCC. The clinical evaluation included relief of pain, range of pronation/supination, and DRUJ stability (**Table 1**). We also analyzed the relationship between the clinical result and the time from the initial injury, and between the clinical result and ulnar variance, in both groups.

RESULTS

After a foveal repair of the TFCC, 15 among 24 wrists had no pain in the arthroscopic group, and 60 among 66 wrists indicated no pain in the open group. Severe pain remained in 2 wrists in the

Table 1
DRUJ evaluating system

		Points
Pain	Severe (always painful)	0
	Moderate (pain in motion or twisting)	1
	Mild (occasionally painful)	2
	No pain	4
Range of pronation/ supination	<100°	0
	100–119°	1
	120–139°	2
	140–159°	3
	More than 159°	4
DRUJ stability	++ (no end point in any direction)	0
	+ (at least 1 end point either in dorsal or palmar)	1
	± (looser than intact contralateral side)	2
	− (stable DRUJ)	4

Points for each category were added and evaluated as:

Excellent: 11–12 points

Good: 9–10 points

Fair: 6–8 points

Poor: 0–5 points

arthroscopic group and in 2 wrists in the open group. In 4 wrists in the arthroscopic group, pain recurred at 8 to 12 months after the surgery. There was no loss of range of rotation before surgery, but 1 wrist showed a 45-degree loss of supination after surgery in each group. DRUJ instability was found in all wrists before surgery. There was no postoperative DRUJ instability in 17 wrists in the arthroscopic group and 56 wrists in the open group, respectively. Moderate to severe DRUJ instability was noted in 7 wrists in the arthroscopic repair group and 4 wrists following an open repair.

The final clinical results obtained were 13 excellent, 3 good, 4 fair, and 4 poor in the arthroscopic group, and 56 excellent, 6 good, 2 fair, and 2 poor in the open group. In the arthroscopic group, the acute and subacute injured cases achieved excellent clinical results. Cases with excellent and good results had surgery within 7 months of the injury (average 4 months). Cases with fair and poor clinical results had an arthroscopic repair at an average of 19 months after the initial injury (range 7 months to 4 years). In patients with a +2-mm positive ulnar variance, there were 1 excellent, 2 fair, and 2 poor results. The patient with a neutral to −1-mm variance wrist obtained 12 excellent, 3 good, 2 fair,

and 2 poor clinical results. There were no differences in the clinical results in the acute, subacute, and chronic cases in the open repair group.

SUMMARY

We have found the techniques described in this article, the arthroscopic transosseous repair of the TFCC and the open transosseous repair of the TFCC to the fovea, to be reliable and successful in treating patients with a foveal disruption of the TFCC with DRUJ instability. Both techniques represent anatomic repair of the RUL, which is nearly vertical from the fovea.

We obtained excellent clinical results with the arthroscopic transosseous repair technique, which reattaches the TFCC into the fovea directly. Excellent clinical results were also obtained in acute and subacute cases, which were treated within 7 months. However, chronic cases 7 months after the initial injury achieved only fair and poor clinical results. This difference may be caused by the healing capacity of the detached site of the TFCC, or because an arthroscopic debridement of the detached site of the TFCC at the fovea was difficult compared with the open repair technique. Another possible cause could be cutting out of the sutures from the TFC in chronic cases. We also found only fair clinical results in the positive ulnar variance cases. When the ulna shows a positive variance, the sutured site was subjected to higher loads from the ulnar head during forearm rotation compared with neutral or minus variance wrists. I prefer the arthroscopic repair method. If the fovea and the DRUJ are poorly visualized at the time of DRUJ arthroscopy, or if the TFCC is in poor condition, prohibiting an arthroscopic repair, then I switch to the open procedure and reconstruct the TFCC with other methods. An arthroscopic transosseous repair is not suitable for excessive ulnar positive variance, so I now consider more than +2 mm of ulnar variance to be a contraindication to the arthroscopic procedure, and I now proceed with an open repair and ulnar shortening or wafer resection.

We obtained excellent clinical results with an open repair technique in foveal detachment of the TFCC in fresh, subacute, and chronic cases. It provided pain relief while restoring a stable DRUJ without a loss of forearm rotation. Direct visualization of the fovea assures a successful repair the TFCC in subacute and chronic cases.

REFERENCES

1. Palmer AK, Werner FW. The triangular fibrocartilage complex of the wrist - anatomy and function. J Hand Surg 1981;6:153–62.

2. Nakamura T, Yabe Y, Horiuchi Y. Functional anatomy of the triangular fibrocartilage complex. J Hand Surg Br 1996;21:581–6.

3. Makita A, Nakamura T, Takayama S, et al. The shape of the triangular fibrocartilage during forearm rotation. J Hand Surg Br 2003;28:537–45.

4. Palmer AK, Werner FW. Biomechanics of the distal radioulnar joint. Clin Orthop 1984;187:26–35.

5. Nakamura T, Makita A. The proximal ligamentous component of the triangular fibrocartilage complex: functional anatomy and three-dimensional changes in length of the radioulnar ligament during pronation-supination. J Hand Surg Br 2000;25:479–86.

6. Spinner M, Kaplan EB. Extensor carpi ulnaris. Its relationship to the stability of the distal radioulnar joint. Clin Orthop 1970;68:124–9.

7. Nakamura T, Yabe Y. Histological anatomy of the triangular fibrocartilage complex of the human wrist. Ann Anat 2000;182:567–72.

8. Nakamura T, Yabe Y, Horiuchi Y, et al. Origins and insertions of the triangular fibrocartilage complex – A histological study. J Hand Surg Br 2001;26:446–54.

9. Palmer AK. Triangular fibrocartilage complex lesions: a classification. J Hand Surg Am 1989;14: 594–606.

10. Haugstvedt JR, Berger RA, Nakamura T, et al. Relative contributions of the ulnar attachment of the triangular fibrocartilage complex to the dynamic stability of the distal radioulnar joint. J Hand Surg 2006;26A: 445–51.

11. Atzei A. Arthroscopic management of DRUJ instability following TFCC ulnar tears. In: del Pinal F, Mathoulin C, Luchetti R, editors. Arthroscopic management of distal radius fractures. Berlin: Springer; 2010. p. 73–88.

12. Manami A, Kato H. Ulnar shortening for triangular fibrocartilage complex tears associated with ulnar positive variance. J Hand Surg Am 1998;23:904–8.

13. Nakamura T, Yabe Y, Horiuchi Y, et al. Ulnar shortening procedure for the ulnocarpal and distal radioulnar joints disorders. J Jap Soc Surg Hand 1998; 15:119–26.

14. Nishiwaki M, Nakamura T, Nakao Y, et al. Ulnar shortening effect on the distal radioulnar stability: a biomechanical study. J Hand Surg Am 2005;30: 719–26.

15. Nishiwaki M, Nakamura T, Nagura T, et al. Ulnar shortening effect on the distal radioulnar joint pressure: a biomechanical study. J Hand Surg Am 2007;33:198–205.

16. Trumble TE, Vedder N. Isolated tears of the triangular fibrocartilage: management by early arthroscopic repair. J Hand Surg Am 1997;22:57–65.

17. Haugstvedt JR, Husby T. Results of repair of peripheral tears in the triangular fibrocartilage complex using an arthroscopic suture technique. Scan J Plast Reconstr Surg 1999;33:439–47.

18. Millants P, De Smet L, Van Ransbeeck H. Outcome study of arthroscopic suturing of ulnar avulsion of the triangular fibrocartilage complex of the wrist. Chir Main 2002;21:298–300.

19. Lindau T, Adlercreutz C, Aspenberg P. Peripheral tears of the triangular fibrocartilage complex cause distal radioulnar joint instability after distal radius fractures. J Hand Surg Am 2000;25:464–8.

20. Atzei A, Rizzo A, Luchetti R, et al. Arthroscopic foveal repair of triangular fibrocartilage complex peripheral lesion with distal radioulnar joint instability. Tech Hand Upper Extrem Surg 2008;12:226–35.

21. Iwasaki N, Minami A. Arthroscopically assisted reattachment of avulsed triangular fibrocartilage complex to the fovea of the ulnar head. J Hand Surg Am 2009;34:1323–6.

22. Hermansdorfer JD, Kleinman WB. Management of chronic peripheral tears of the triangular fibrocartilage complex. J Hand Surg Am 1991;16:340–6.

23. Sennward GR, Lauterburg M, Zdravkovic V. A new technique of reattachment after traumatic avulsion of the TFCC at its ulnar insertion. J Hand Surg Br 1995;20:178–84.

24. Chou KH, Sarris IK, Sotereanos DG. Suture anchor repair of ulnar sided triangular fibrocartilage complex tears. J Hand Surg Br 2003;28:546–50.

25. Walker LG. Stabilization of the distal radioulnar joint after ulnar styloid nonunion using Mitek anchors. Orthop Review 1994;23:769–72.

26. Nakamura T, Nakao Y, Ikegami H, et al. Open repair of the ulnar disruption of the triangular fibrocartilage complex with double 3D-mattress suturing technique. Tech Upper Extrem Surg 2004;8:116–23.

27. Tay SC, Tomita K, Berger RA. The "ulnar fovea sign" for defining ulnar wrist pain: an analysis of sensitivity and specificity. J Hand Surg Am 2007;32:438–44.

28. Moriya T, Aoki M, Iba K, et al. Effect of triangular ligament tears on distal radioulnar joint instability and evaluation of three clinical tests: a biomechanical study. J Hand Surg Eur 2009;34:219–23.

29. Nakamura T, Yabe Y, Horiuchi Y. Fat-suppression magnetic resonance imaging of the triangular fibrocartilage complex – comparison with spin echo, gradient echo pulse sequence and histology. J Hand Surg Br 1999;24:22–6.

30. Tanaka T, Yoshioka H, Ueno T, et al. Comparison between high-resolution MRI with a microscopy coil and arthroscopy in triangular fibrocartilage complex injury. J Hand Surg Am 2006;31:1308–14.

Minimal Invasive Management of Scaphoid Fractures: From Fresh to Nonunion

W.Y. Clara Wong, MBChB, MRCS, FRCSEd (Orth), FHKAM (Orthopaedic Surgery), FHKCOS, P.C. Ho, MBBS, FRCS(Edinburgh), FHKCOS, FHKAM(Orthopaedic Surgery)*

KEYWORDS

- Scaphoid fracture • Nonunion • Surgical technique
- Arthroscopy

SCAPHOID FRACTURE MANAGEMENT OVERVIEW

Scaphoid fracture is the most common carpal fracture.[1,2] It accounts for approximately 60% to 90% of carpal fractures and 11% of hand fractures.[1,3,4]

The term "scaphoid" is derived from the Greek word "skaphē," which means skiff and is named for its likeness to a boat. However, the 3-dimensional shape of the scaphoid is more complex. The precise evaluation of the fracture configuration, angulation, displacement, and accuracy of screw placement is hindered by the peculiar twisted peanutlike shape of the scaphoid.[5–7] Besides its shape, the scaphoid is predominantly articular.[8,9] Preservation of the articular congruity is just as important as with the treatment of any articular fracture. With the predominantly articular nature of the scaphoid, there are few potential sites for the entrance of perforating vessels. It is well known that scaphoid has a tenuous vascular supply.[10,11] Complications of delayed union, nonunion, and avascular necrosis are not uncommon. Moreover, the scaphoid is the focus of ligamentous attachment. It is the key link of the wrist and governs the carpal kinematics.[12,13] Therefore, preservation of the scaphoid anatomy and vascularity is critical for normal hand and wrist function.

Most (>80%) patients who sustain scaphoid fractures are young men between the ages of 20 and 30 years.[3] These patients are active with high functional demands; hence, prolonged cast immobilization comes at some cost, which includes wrist stiffness, decreased grip strength, a significant rehabilitation period, and physical and economic morbidity.[14–18] Percutaneous screw fixation is currently practiced. We have been using percutaneous fixation for acute scaphoid fractures since 1991.[19–21] Excellent and reliable results are frequently obtained.[19–24]

Scaphoid nonunion continues to present a unique clinical challenge. Natural history studies by Mark and colleagues,[25] Ruby and colleagues,[26] and Linstrom and Nystrom[27] indicated an incidence of almost 100% of radiographic wrist arthritis between 5 and 20 years after scaphoid nonunion in symptomatic patients. Because most scaphoid nonunions occur in young and active individuals, the development of scaphoid nonunion advanced collapse (SNAC) changes poses

Department of Orthopaedics and Traumatology, Prince of Wales Hospital, 30-32 Ngan Shing Street, Shatin, N.T., Hong Kong
* Corresponding author.
E-mail address: pcho@ort.cuhk.edu.hk

Hand Clin 27 (2011) 291–307
doi:10.1016/j.hcl.2011.06.003
0749-0712/11/$ – see front matter © 2011 Published by Elsevier Inc.

a significant threat to their normal wrist and upper limb function. Timely surgical intervention, by anatomic restoration of a stable scaphoid architecture and its linkage to adjacent bones, is the goal before arthritis sets in. With the advancement of arthroscopic techniques and its advantages of minimal surgical trauma to the scaphoid blood supply and its ligamentous connections, arthroscopic bone grafting (ABG) provides a favorable environment for healing scaphoid nonunion. ABG has become our primary treatment in all noncomplicated scaphoid delayed unions and nonunions.

ACUTE SCAPHOID FRACTURE
Classification

Classifying scaphoid fractures by dividing the scaphoid into thirds according to its length is simple and easy to understand, but the distinct groups of fracture at the tuberosity, distal articular surface, and proximal pole of the scaphoid are neglected. The Mayo classification for scaphoid fractures is commonly used in clinical practice and can address these distinct fracture groups.[28] However, the exact level of distal one-third, middle one-third, waist, and proximal one-third fractures is arbitrary, which produces limited interobserver and intraobserver reliability. Herbert devised a classification system that combines fracture anatomy, stability, and chronicity of injury.[29,30] This system provides a helpful rationale for treatment options and prognostic value. Similarly, fractures through the body are not clearly addressed. With only the distal oblique fracture in type B1 or waist fracture in type B2, the true fracture pattern and level in scaphoid body cannot be well represented.

Compson and colleagues[7,31–33] identified 3 basic fracture patterns involving the body of the scaphoid: a transverse waist fracture, a sulcal fracture, and a proximal pole fracture. The scaphoid waist is the narrowest part and at the midportion of the bone. A transverse waist fracture lies roughly perpendicular to the long axis of the scaphoid and across the narrowest midportion. A sulcal fracture (Fig. 1A), probably the most common scaphoid fracture according to Compson, is oblique to its long axis, starts from the region close to the origin of the dorsal scapholunate (SL) ligament, along the dorsal ridge, to the lateral apex of the ridge and crosses the palmar face to the scaphocapitate (SC) facet. At the lateral apex of the dorsal ridge, there are 3 variations (see Fig. 1B): the fracture line passes proximally, distally, or on both sides of the apex. The butterfly fragment in the third variation is a kind of fracture comminution (see Fig. 1C). A proximal pole fracture runs from under the attachment of the dorsal

SL ligament, proximal to the dorsal ridge, and crosses the radioscaphoid joint to the proximal end of the SC joint.

To categorize the fractures occurring in the scaphoid body and the distinct groups, we propose a new classification system that can accommodate all the scaphoid fracture patterns (Fig. 2). To delineate the fracture pattern, a scaphoid radiograph series should include a posteroanterior (PA) view, a lateral view, a PA with ulnar deviation, a PA with ulnar deviation with 20° angulation of the x-ray beam angled toward the elbow, a semipronated view, and a semisupinated view. The scaphoid body and its long axis is best visualized in the PA view with ulnar deviation and 20° angulation, in which the x-ray is projected perpendicular to the plane of the scaphoid body. A semipronated view provides the clearest view to visualize a sulcal fracture and differentiates it from a transverse waist fracture.

We would like to define the scaphoid body as the portion articulating with the capitate. A type B body fracture is divided into the distal one-third (type B1), middle one-third (type B2), proximal one-third (type B3), and sulcal (type B4) fractures. The third is defined by dividing the SC facet into 3 equal portions in the scaphoid view. The distinct fracture groups include type A (distal pole fracture), type A1 (scaphoid tubercle fracture), type A2 (distal articular fracture), and type C (proximal pole fracture), in which any fracture line that passes beyond the SC facet in the proximal part of scaphoid falls into type C scaphoid fracture. Transscaphoid perilunate fracture dislocation is classified as type D.

A displaced fracture is defined as a fracture gap greater than 1 mm, a fracture step greater than 1 mm, an SL angle greater than 60°, a radiolunate (RL) angle greater than 15°,[18] a lateral intrascaphoid angle greater than 45°, or an anteroposterior (AP) intrascaphoid angle greater than 35°.[34]

Authors' Experience

A retrospective review on all the operated acute or subacute scaphoid fractures in our hospital over about a 5-year period was conducted. From August 2005 to June 2010, 91 operations were performed for acute and subacute scaphoid fractures. There were 79 men and 12 women with an average age of 28 years (range, 13–60 years). The right scaphoid was fractured in 34 patients and the left in 57 patients; 19 of them were smokers. All fractures were grouped according to our classification (see Fig. 2). Forty-six fractures were type B2 (middle one-third), 26 were type B4 (sulcal fracture), 7 were type C (proximal pole), 6 were type D (transscaphoid perilunate fracture

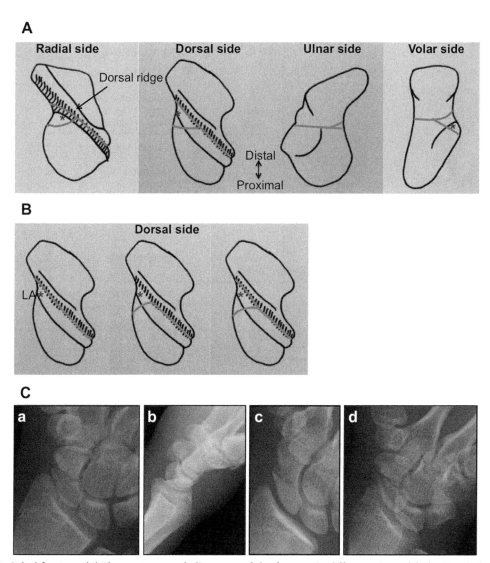

Fig. 1. Sulcal fracture. (*A*) The anatomy and alignment of the fracture in different views. (*B*) The 3 variations on a dorsal view (lateral apex of the dorsal ridge [*asterisk*]). (*C*) Example of a sulcal fracture of the third variation with a butterfly fragment. (a) PA view. (b) Lateral view. (c) PA view with ulnar deviation. (d) Semipronation view. (*Data from* Compson JP. The anatomy of acute scaphoid fractures. A three-dimensional analysis of patterns. J Bone Joint Surg Br 1998;80:218–24.)

dislocation), 5 were type B3 (proximal one-third), and 1 was a type B1 (distal one-third). Ten patients had a concomitant upper limb injury, including 5 distal radius fractures, 1 radial head fracture, 1 olecranon fracture, 1 complex elbow fracture dislocation, and 2 radial and ulnar shaft fractures. There were 23 displaced scaphoid fractures. Fracture comminution was identified in 50 patients, in whom more than 2 bony fragments were identified radiographically. In these 91 scaphoid fractures, 15 patients had a delayed presentation from 3 weeks to 7 months after the injury; 4 were displaced fractures.

Most operations (71 patients) were performed under general anesthesia, 9 under plexus anesthesia, 7 under intravenous local anesthesia, and 4 under local anesthesia.

We have been using a volar approach for percutaneous screw fixation since 1991.[19–21] For the displaced acute fractures (19 cases), a closed reduction was performed first. Fifteen fractures were successfully reduced by closed means, whereas 4 fractures needed an arthroscopic-assisted reduction. For comminuted acute fractures (44 cases), the fracture gap was assessed fluoroscopically and arthroscopically. Wrist arthroscopy was

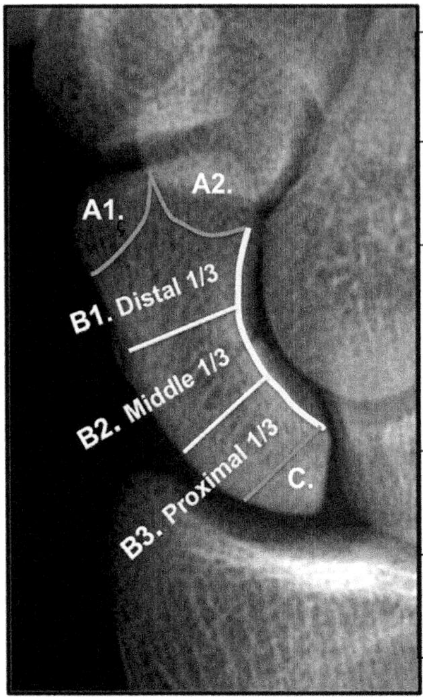

Ho & Wong's Classification of Scaphoid Fracture			No. of Patients in our series
A (Distal Pole)	1	Scaphoid Tubercle	0
	2	Distal Articular	0
B (Body)	1	Distal 1/3	1
	2	Middle 1/3	46
	3	Proximal 1/3	5
	4	Sulcal Fracture	26
C (Proximal Pole)		Proximal Pole	7
D		Trans-scaphoid Perilunate Fracture Dislocation	6

Fig. 2. Eight scaphoid fracture types in Ho and Wong's classification of scaphoid fracture.

performed when there was a clinical suspicion of an associated intraarticular injury such as a triangular fibrocartilage complex (TFCC) tear, SL dissociation, or an osteochondral lesion. A total of 29 arthroscopies were performed in these acute fractures; 5 patients underwent pinning for SL dissociation, 5 underwent LT (lunotriquetral) pinning for LT dissociation, and 7 received arthroscopic treatment of a TFCC tear, and a bone graft was inserted in 3 cases.[35]

For the 15 fractures with delayed presentation, arthroscopy was performed to assess the fracture alignment, stability, and healing status to determine the treatment methods, which included splinting alone (6 cases), screw fixation (5 cases), and Kirschner wire (K-wire) fixation (4 cases). Among the fixation group, 6 cases required ABG.

Surgical Technique

Percutaneous screw fixation can be performed under general anesthesia, plexus anesthesia, or intravenous local anesthesia. The patient is placed supine; the arm is abducted 70° and placed on the arm board. Excessive shoulder abduction may cause difficulty in passively pronating the forearm to facilitate the guide pin reduction process. Use of a tourniquet is optional, and the tourniquet is usually placed over the arm as a standby. After sterile draping, there should be sufficient room for easy rotation of the forearm during the procedure.

Good-quality fluoroscopy is essential to confirm the fracture alignment and hardware position. The fluoroscope is positioned over the arm board, directly over the wrist, vertical to the floor at the highest magnification.

Five views are mandatory during the procedure to assess the fracture alignment, guide pin, and screw position: AP, lateral, scaphoid (AP ulnar deviation), semisupination, and semipronation views. The semisupination view (**Fig. 3**) is used to assess the correct position of the guide pin because this view gives the best spatial relationship of the guide pin with the proximal pole, distal pole, and dorsal and volar borders of the scaphoid. For a normal scaphoid, this alignment appears bean shaped in the semisupination view. We call this the bean view. The ulnovolar border of the scaphoid appears a bit concave; the dorsoradial border of the scaphoid is C-shaped, with the dorsal tuberosity at the midpart of the C, that is, the scaphoid dorsal ridge. The midportion of the bean is the sharp turn between the proximal and distal parts of the scaphoid. The distal end of the bean represents the distal pole of the scaphoid, whereas the proximal end of the bean represents the proximal pole of the scaphoid. The semipronation view, with some ulnar deviation of the wrist, demonstrates the longest axis of the scaphoid

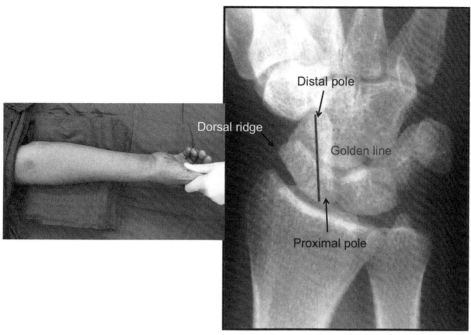

Fig. 3. Semisupination view/bean view. The arm is 90° abducted, the elbow extended, and the forearm 45° supinated. The proximal forearm is elevated with a folded towel. Avoid placing it underneath the wrist to dazzle the imaging intensity. The golden line, landmark, and position of the guide pin as shown in the bean view.

and the concave inner articulating surface of the scaphoid with the capitate.

Correct alignment should be confirmed with these 5 views such that no step is present. Some gapping can usually be corrected after screw compression.

The scaphoid tends to rotate into flexion and pronation with loading.[36,37] With a fracture to the waist of the scaphoid, the distal scaphoid rotates around the radioscaphocapitate ligament into an abnormal flexion, ulnar deviation, and pronation posture. The lunate and the attached proximal part of the scaphoid rotate into an abnormal extension, supination, and radial deviation.[37–41] Therefore, the capitolunate (CL) angle, RL angle, and lunocapitate angle should also be assessed to detect any humpback deformity of the scaphoid and dorsal intercalated segment instability (DISI) alignment.

Closed Reduction

Closed reduction is performed with the forearm placed on a folded towel (**Fig. 4**). Traction is applied by grasping the thumb, and the wrist is extended and ulnar deviated, with forearm in full supination or slight hypersupination, which reduces the humpback deformity. Traction also opens up the radiovolar interval between the scaphoid and the trapezium and improves access

for guide pin insertion. The traction force helps to improve any step off through ligamentotaxis.

In the presence of a DISI deformity and extended lunate, the deformity can be corrected first before realigning the distal part of the scaphoid to the proximal one. It is achieved by flexing the wrist to restore the normal RL and CL angles. The lunate is then temporarily transfixed with a 1.1-mm K-wire inserted from the dorsal distal radius through a mini-incision. To minimize the risk of entrapping the extensor tendons, we adjust the pneumatic drill to an oscillating mode.

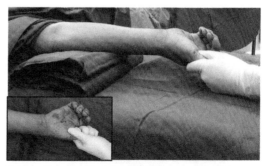

Fig. 4. Close reduction technique. Traction force is applied by grasping the thumb, and the wrist is extended, with forearm in full supination or slight hypersupination.

Correcting the lunate alignment indirectly improves the extension deformity of the proximal part of the scaphoid, provided that the SL ligament is intact, which realigns the distal part of the scaphoid with the proximal part.

Landmarks and Position of the Guide Pin

Correct position of the guide pin determines the screw position. The closer the pin is to the scaphoid axis, the longer the screw that can be used and the better the compression of the fracture.[42,43] There are several landmarks to guide the entry point and direction of the guide pin.

1. The bean view is the most important view to ensure optimal placement of the guide pin, which should pass through the interval between the middle and volar one-third of the bean along its volar border, the Golden line (see **Fig. 3**). If the guide pin does not appear to cut out of the scaphoid on the other views, this represents the longest scaphoid length with maximum bone purchase.

2. Hung advocated tracing the direction of the K-wire on the skin with a marker.[19,20] In the AP view, a K-wire is placed over the skin to produce an overlap image on the scaphoid. A true lateral radiograph is then obtained. The K-wire is again placed over the skin and the position is again marked on the skin. These 2 lines provide references for the direction of the guide pin.

3. The best angle of insertion of the guide pin is 40° to the sagittal plane and 45° to the coronal plane. The entry point should be between the middle of the scaphoid tubercle, and the exit point should be around the distal half of the proximal pole of the scaphoid (**Fig. 5**). This placement provides the maximum purchase of the screw but may be modified according to the fracture type and pattern.[19–21]

Placement of the Guide Pin

A 1.1-mm guide pin is used, but we occasionally use a 1.2-mm K-wire to establish the entry point and then exchange it for a 1.1-mm guide pin.

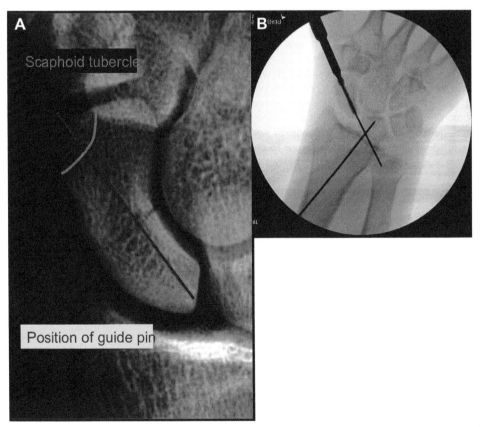

Fig. 5. Landmark and position of the guide pin in scaphoid view. (A) Entry point: middle of the scaphoid tubercle. Exit point: around distal half of proximal pole. (B) Position of the guide pin and the inserting screw. The RL joint was transfixed with a 1.1-mm K-wire to correct the fracture deformity before scaphoid guide pin insertion.

The fracture site must be temporarily transfixed with another smaller-diameter K-wire before taking out the 1.2-mm K-wire, otherwise the fracture alignment will be lost and it will be difficult to reinsert the guide pin along the old tract. Goddard[44] advocated the use of a 12-gauge intravenous needle as a trocar for the guide pin. By levering on the trapezium and by rotating the needle with its bevel facing ulnarly, the distal pole of the scaphoid is brought more radially, which facilitates guide wire insertion.

After the closed reduction, the proper alignment must be confirmed fluoroscopically, the thumb grasped with one hand to maintain the alignment, and the guide pin held with another hand. The site of skin entry is usually 5 mm more distal than the scaphoid tubercle. We prefer to locate the skin entry site first by inserting the guide pin by hand into the scaphotrapezial joint under the AP view and the bean view. The bean view is used to determine the volar dorsal position of the entry site. A 3-mm transverse skin incision is then made along the skin crease. Small pointed-tip scissors are used to perforate the scaphotrapeziotrapezoid (STT) joint, release a hemarthrosis, and dilate the tract to the starting point on the scaphoid tubercle, which is located along the long axis of the scaphoid on the bean view and between the middle and radial third of scaphoid tubercle in the AP view. A small trough is made with the tip of the scissors on the scaphoid tubercle.

The guide pin is then aimed at 40° in the sagittal plane and at 45° in the coronal plane. We find it easier aiming the guide pin toward the Lister tubercle located with the index finger of the surgeon's hand. The position should be checked in all 5 views.

Bone resistance is normally felt when the guide pin approaches the cortex at the exit point. When the guide wire is in a foreshortened position, the exit point is too close to the entry point or this point is too far away from the cortex. This position indicates that the pin is directed too dorsally, hitting the dorsal cortex, and away from the long axis of the scaphoid. This position will not provide adequate fracture fixation and should be readjusted.

With the tip of the guide pin at the opposite cortex, the length of the inserted part is measured. The actual screw length should be 4 mm less than this measured pin length to allow for subsequent fracture compression and sinking of the screw head at the entry point. If an attempt is made to seat the screw by overdriving it against the opposite unreamed cortex, the fracture will be further displaced apart (**Fig. 6**). For Asian women, the usual screw length is about 20 to 24 mm, whereas the length is 22 to 26 mm in men. If the exact pin length is beyond 26 to 30 mm, correct alignment of the pin without protruding out of the cortex must be ensured by repeating all 5 radiographic views.

The guide pin is advanced further after measurement through the opposite cortex and out of skin and secured in place with artery forces. The exit point of the guide pin should always be at the 3-4 arthroscopy portal. Care must be taken to not entrap the extensor tendons. The risk can be minimized with the use of an oscillating mode of the K-wire driver. If the guide pin is accidentally broken inside the wrist during drilling or tapping, it can still be taken out with its exposed part on both the dorsal and volar side of the wrist.

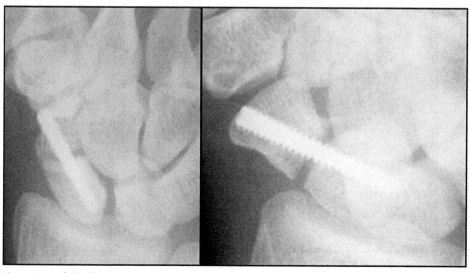

Fig. 6. Distraction of the fracture site when the screw was too long.

After screw placement, all 5 radiographic views should be finally checked to ensure proper position, fracture compression, and no screw protrusion before concluding the surgery. Postoperatively, free mobilization is allowed. A thumb spica brace is offered to high-risk patients, who are older individuals with osteopenic bone, have significant fracture comminution, proximal pole fractures, or are noncompliant. Supervised mobilization exercises out of splint are necessary in these patients.

PROXIMAL ONE-THIRD AND PROXIMAL POLE FRACTURES

A short-tip threaded screw is used in proximal one-third fracture or some proximal pole fractures so that all the threads of the screw tip have crossed the fracture line into the proximal fragment before compression is achieved. If a short-tip threaded screw is not available or the proximal fragment is too small, a cannulated screw can be inserted from the dorsal wrist through the advanced guide pin, which is inserted from the volar wrist (**Fig. 7**).

The technique of guide pin insertion in these fractures is similar, except with the entry point a bit more dorsoradial and aimed volarward in the proximal pole because the proximal pole fragment is wider on the volar aspect.[45]

TRANSSCAPHOID PERILUNATE FRACTURE DISLOCATION

There were 6 patients suffering from transscaphoid perilunate fracture dislocation, with an average age of 26 years. Four patients were men. The left side was affected in 5 patients; 4 were associated with other fractures in the same limb. The scaphoid fractures were fixed with percutaneous screws. Wrist arthroscopy was performed in 3 cases to assess and assist the fracture reduction (**Fig. 8**). Bone graft was performed in 1 patient as a second stage surgery 1 week later. All fractures united in an average of 20.5 weeks, with no avascular necrosis. All patients had nearly full range of wrist motion and good grip power.

DELAYED PRESENTATION

There were 15 patients with delayed presentation at an average of 10 weeks (range, 3–28 weeks) after the injury. The fracture line was still prominent on radiography. Wrist arthroscopies were performed in all of these patients. When the fracture fragments were still mobile with little evidence of healing or in the presence of significant gap and/or step, percutaneous fixation was performed using screws (in 5 patients) or K-wires (in 4 patients), augmented with ABG procedures. When the fracture site was shown to be stable with a bony end

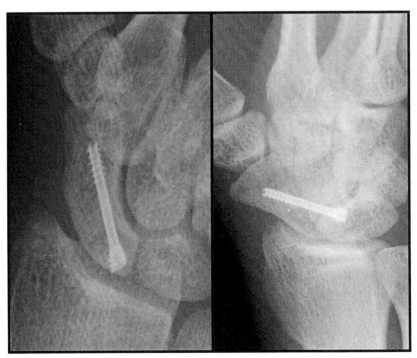

Fig. 7. Screw was inserted along the guide pin in an antegrade direction from the dorsal wrist. The guide pin was inserted in a volar approach. A shorter screw was used in the proximal pole fracture.

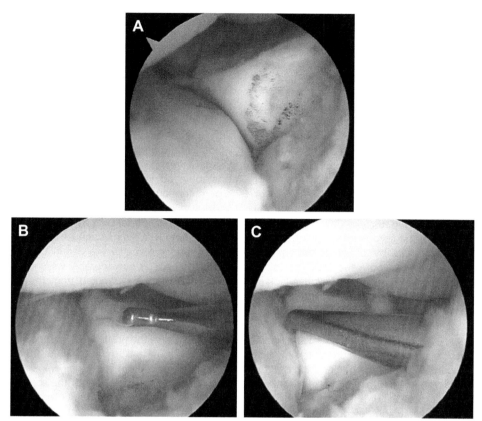

Fig. 8. Midcarpal joint arthroscopy in transscaphoid perilunate fracture dislocation (type D). Viewing at midcarpal ulna portal. (*A*) Rotational deformity at LT joint. (*B*) Reduction with a probe to depress the triquetral. (*C*) Stable LT interval after LT pinning.

point on direct probing, in the absence of a significant gap, step, or DISI deformity, no fixation was performed and external immobilization with casting or splinting was done and maintained for 2 to 8 weeks. Six patients were treated in this manner, and all fractures healed uneventfully.

SCAPHOID NONUNION
ABG

From April 1997 to November 2009, there were 65 men and 4 women presenting with a symptomatic nonunion, with an average age of 27.6 (ranged 14–53). The median duration of the pathology was 10 months (range 4–276). Forty-two patients (60.9%) suffered from sport-related injuries. There were 10 distal third, 31 mid-third and 28 proximal third fractures. Twenty cases (29%) showed DISI deformity radiologically.

Surgical Technique

Patient is placed supine with the operated arm suspended on a traction tower. Adrenaline, 1 in 200,000 dilution, is injected in the portal site skin and capsule

to reduce bleeding. We perform a routine inspection of both the radiocarpal joint through the 3-4 portal and midcarpal joint through the midcarpal radial (MCR) portal using a 2.7-mm video arthroscope. Any accompanying chondral lesion related to SNAC wrist changes should be documented since it may affect the prognosis and choice of procedure. The fracture site cannot be seen from the radiocarpal joint unless it is very proximal. It is frequently embedded within the reflection of the joint capsule. This fact is also important because the capsular reflection frequently helps to contain the bone graft, which is implanted from the midcarpal joint from a distal to proximal direction. We perform bone grafting through the midcarpal joint portals in all cases because it provides the most convenient and direct approach to the nonunion site.

Bone Grafting in the Presence of Previous Internal Fixation

In the midcarpal joint, we generally select the midcarpal ulna as the entry portal and the MCR as the working portal. Two accessory portals may also be recruited. The triquetrohamate portal is most useful for outflow and is located by palpating the extensor carpi ulnaris (ECU) tendon and moving distally until the palpating finger reaches the hamate bone. This portal is then located at the axilla between the ECU tendon and the hamate. The STT portal is situated about 1 cm radial and slightly distal to the MCR portal, just ulnar to the extensor pollicis longus (EPL) tendon, at the junction between the scaphoid, trapezoid, and trapezium. Care should be taken to avoid injury to the radial artery, which is radial to the EPL tendon.

The nonunion site is located by the presence of a cleavage line in the scaphoid articular surface or with frank articular cartilage disruption and fibrous tissue interposition (**Fig. 9**).

The firmness of the fibrous interposition should be assessed carefully by direct palpation with a small probe inserted from the MCR portal. A stable fibrous fixation explains the relative lack of symptoms in some patients. In delayed union, the fibrous tissue may cover the bridging callus, which usually forms in the central part of the fracture. If stable bony tissue is appreciated after initial debridement of the overlying fibrous tissue, one needs to reconsider whether bone grafting is actually necessary because this may represent an ongoing healing process. If a frank bony defect is encountered, the cartilage defect is then enlarged with a suction punch to improve access to the nonunion cavity. Curettage of the nonunion site with a fine-angled curette, motorized 2.0- or 2.9-mm shaver, and 2.9- or 3.5-mm burr is then performed until all the fibrous scar tissue and sclerotic bone have been removed and the implant is exposed. The frequently intact cartilage over the proximal side of the nonunion site or any pseudocapsule should be preserved as much as possible to avoid subsequent graft spillage to the radiocarpal joint. Both ends of the nonunion site are burred

until healthy-looking cancellous bone with punctate bleeding is seen (**Fig. 10**).

We find it unnecessary to inflate the tourniquet during this procedure, which helps to determine the vascularity of the remaining bone fragments. Further curettage of the proximal fragment until healthy punctate bleeding can be continued by switching the instrument to the STT portal if necessary. Implant stability is then assessed visually with manipulation and, if necessary, using a C-arm image intensifier. If the compression screw is unstable and loose, it can be exchanged with a percutaneous technique.

An arthroscopic cannula is introduced through an appropriate portal directly opposing the fracture defect. A 3.2-mm cannula can be inserted initially and replaced by a 5-mm cannula when the joint space is considerably widened. Cancellous bone graft is harvested from the iliac crest using either trephine or open technique through a small incision. The volume of the bone graft obtained has to be at least 3 to 5 times that of the defect because the graft needs to be compressed tightly in the defect to increase its strength. The bone graft is then cut into small chips using scissors and delivered through the cannula with a slightly undersized trocar such as bone biopsy trocar (**Fig. 11**).

The most proximal and dorsal part of the defect needs to be meticulously filled up first. Fluoroscopy is helpful to confirm the completeness and adequacy of the graft filling. A small depressor can be used at intervals to mold and contour the graft to the articular surface of the scaphoid (**Fig. 12**). Complete filling of the defect and satisfactory scaphoid alignment is then confirmed fluoroscopically (**Figs. 13** and **14**).

At the end of the procedure, marrow clot taken from the iliac crest can be injected into the graft

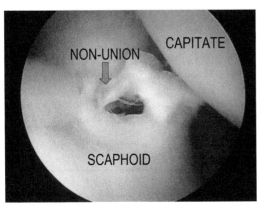

Fig. 9. Frank articular cartilage disruption and fibrous tissue interposition.

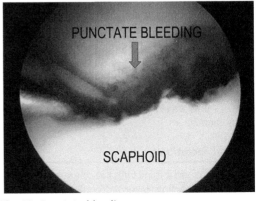

Fig. 10. Punctate bleeding.

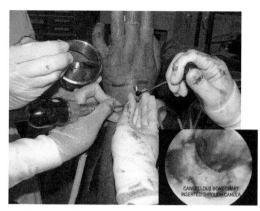

Fig. 11. Bone biopsy trocar.

region to improve osteogenesis and bone healing. We routinely inject 1 mL of fibrin glue on the surface of the graft substance after suctioning any excess fluid to contain the graft in place and to prevent adhesion of the graft to the capitate articular surface, which in some cases may lead to loss of motion at the midcarpal joint.

Bone Grafting Without Previous Internal Fixation

In the midcarpal joint, the nonunion site is identified and managed as previously described. The MCR portal is usually the best portal to take down the fibrosis around the nonunion in the proximal and waist portion. In distal third nonunion, the STT portal is frequently required. After adequate debridement and curettage, the 2 fragments of the nonunion should be mobile enough for subsequent reduction. Any humpback and DISI deformity should be identified (**Fig. 15**).

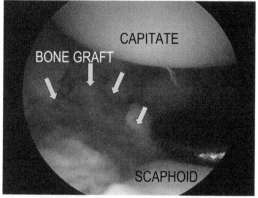

Fig. 12. Graft contouring to the articular surface of the scaphoid.

1. Correction the deformity can be facilitated by the following measures, similar to the reduction of acute scaphoid fracture: In the presence of intact SL ligament, dorsiflexion deformity of proximal pole of scaphoid is corrected by firstly passive wrist flexion to realign the extended lunate with the radius (ie, to restore the normal RL angle). The RL joint is then temporarily transfixed with a percutaneous 1.1 mm K-wire inserted from dorsal distal radius (**Fig. 16**).
2. By traction and manipulation with gentle passive ulnar deviation, hypersupination and extension of the wrist, the distal fragment can be realigned to the proximal one (**Fig. 17**).
3. In distal third nonunion where manipulation of the distal fragment is more difficult, a 1.6 mm K-wire can be inserted through trapezium into the distal fragment of scaphoid for better manipulation.
4. Manipulation of fragment can also be done from within joint using a probe and percutaneous K-wire as joystick.

The fracture can be fixed percutaneously with K-wire inserted either from scaphoid tubercle retrogradely for waist or distal portion nonunion, or from proximal pole antegradely for proximal pole nonunion. Cancellous bone graft is then packed into the nonunion site as previously described to allow better filling of the cavity. When the cavity is half filled, a percutaneous screw can be inserted along the guide pin after predrilling the track. Slight compression of the fracture can usually be achieved. Overcompression may collapse the nonunion site. If the fragment is too small for any screw fixation, multiple K-wires should be used for definitive fixation. We routinely use three 1.1-mm K-wires. Transfixing the SL and SC joints should also be considered for an unstable nonunion. We have used a 2.7-mm BOLD cannulated screw (NewDeal SA, France) for nonunion of the waist and multiple K-wire fixation for distal or proximal nonunion.

After screw insertion, additional bone graft is impacted into the nonunion. When K-wires are used for definitive fixation, the remaining 2 wires can be inserted after completion of the grafting process and are kept in place for up to 10 to 12 weeks.

The wound is approximated with Steri-strips and no stitching is required (**Figs. 18** and **19**).

In cases with early SNAC changes involving the radial styloid and distal scaphoid fragment, fixation of the nonunion is not contraindicated, provided that an adequate radial styloidectomy is done at the same setting to reduce the subsequent impingement.

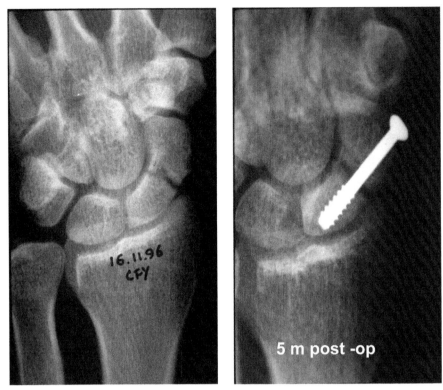

Fig. 13. Scaphoid nonunion 5 months after screw fixation for acute fracture.

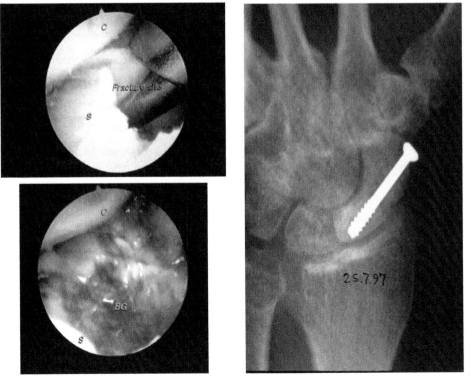

Fig. 14. ABG and result.

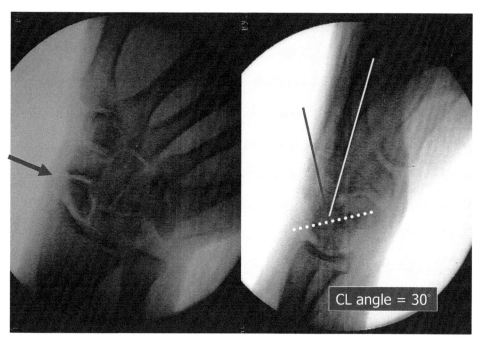

Fig. 15. Increased CL angle in scaphoid nonunion.

Postoperative Care

The plaster slab is maintained for 2 weeks. In cases with DISI deformity, the transfixing pin across the RL joint should be removed by 2 weeks.

Delayed removal may result in iatrogenic breakage of the pin. A below-elbow splint is then fabricated to provide protection to the nonunion site. Active mobilization of the wrist under the supervision of a hand therapist can be initiated as early as 2

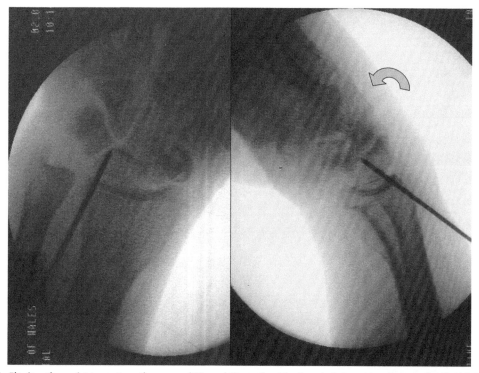

Fig. 16. Flexing the wrist to restore the normal RL and CL angles. The lunate is temporarily transfixed with K-wire.

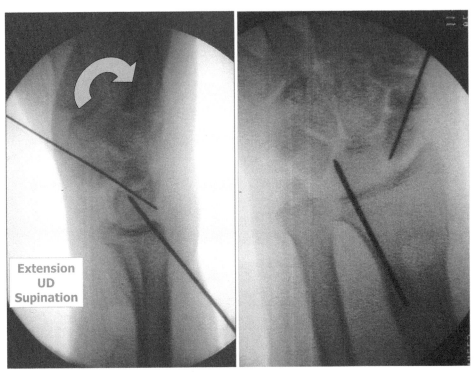

Fig. 17. Extension, ulnar deviation, and supination of the wrist help to realign the distal part of the scaphoid to the proximal one.

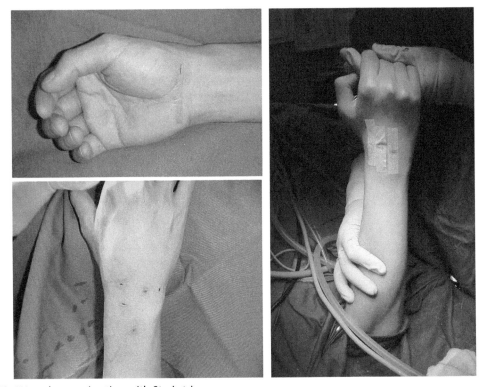

Fig. 18. Wound approximation with Steri-strips.

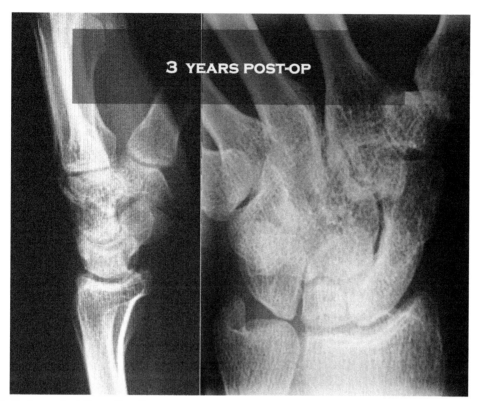

Fig. 19. Radiograph at 6 months after surgery.

weeks after surgery if the nonunion fixation is thought to be stable. This also applies to cases with K-wire fixation. Once clinical union is confirmed, the K-wires can be removed under local anesthesia, typically at week 10 to 12 postoperatively, followed by passive mobilization and then strengthening exercise.

RESULTS OF ABG

In all cases, the procedure was accomplished arthroscopically without reverting to open surgery. The mean operation time was 190 minutes (range,

90–300 minutes). The average follow-up of the remaining 68 cases was 39.5 months (range, 5–125 months). The overall union rate was 91.2% (62/68), including 7 cases of delayed union at 4 to 6 months. The average radiologic union time was 12 weeks (range, 6–39 weeks). Correlation of union status and vascularity of the proximal scaphoid fragment is shown in **Table 1**. Poor intraoperative bleeding of the proximal scaphoid still permitted union in 16 out of 19 cases (84.2%), while good bleeding predicted union in 40 out of 42 cases (95.2%). There were 6 failures in our series. Four patients received further surgery.

Table 1
Correlation of union status and vascularity of proximal scaphoid fragment

Number of Patients in Different Degree of Vascularity of Proximal Scaphoid Fragment			Final Union Status after ABG (Number of Patients)
Good	Fair	Poor	
37	6	12	Union (55)
3	0	4	Delayed Union (7)
2	1	3	Non-union (6)

CONCLUSION

Scaphoid fracture is a common injury to be encountered in our daily practice. Preservation of its anatomy, adjacent ligamentous architecture and vascularity is crucial in the management. This can be achieved with skilful mastering of both the volar approach and arthroscopic techniques, no matter which fracture type and pattern, time of presentation, or associated injury. The development of arthroscopies brings a significant breakthrough in the history of wrist surgeries. It has a definite role in managing difficult scaphoid fracture, delayed union and nonunion. It provides a thorough wrist assessment, comprehensive approach for scaphoid fracture and its sequelae in a minimally invasive manner, a favorable biological environment for the fracture union, and minimal surgical trauma to the ligamentous architecture and vascularity. With the successful results and experience in scaphoid fracture throughout the years, more wrist surgeries can certainly be benefited from this minimal invasive approach, even for the salvage situations.

REFERENCES

1. Kozin SH. Incidence, mechanism, and natural history of scaphoid fractures. Hand Clin 2001;17:515–24.
2. Phillips TG, Reibach AM, Slomiany WP. Diagnosis and management of scaphoid fractures. Am Fam Physician 2004;70:879–84.
3. Hove LM. Epidemiology of scaphoid fractures in Bergen, Norway. Scand J Plast Reconstr Surg Hand Surg 1999;33:423–6.
4. Rhemrev SJ, van Leerdam RH, Ootes D, et al. Non-operative treatment of non-displaced scaphoid fractures may be preferred. Injury 2009;40(6):638–41.
5. Ring D, Jupiter JB, Herndon JH. Acute fractures of the scaphoid. J Am Acad Orthop Surg 2000;8:225–31.
6. Gelberman RH, Wolock BS, Siegel DB. Fractures and non-unions of the carpal scaphoid. J Bone Joint Surg Am 1989;71:1560–5.
7. Compson JP. The anatomy of acute scaphoid fractures. A three-dimensional analysis of patterns. J Bone Joint Surg Br 1998;80:218–24.
8. Jupiter JB, Shin AY, Trumble TE, et al. Traumatic and reconstructive problems of the scaphoid. Instr Course Lect 2001;50:105–22.
9. Berger RA. The anatomy of the scaphoid. Hand Clin 2001;17(4):525–32.
10. Taleisnik J, Kelly PJ. The extraosseous and intraosseous blood supply of the scaphoid bone. J Bone Joint Surg Am 1966;48:1125–37.
11. Gelberman RH, Menon J. The vascularity of the scaphoid bone. J Hand Surg Am 1980;5(5):508–13.
12. Berger RA, Crowninshield RD, Flatt AE. The three-dimensional rotational behaviours of the carpal bones. Clin Orthop 1982;167:303–10.
13. Short WH, Werner FW, Fortino MD, et al. Analysis of the kinematics of the scaphoid and lunate in the intact wrist joint. Hand Clin 1997;13(1):93–108.
14. Bond CD, Shin AY, McBride MT, et al. Percutaneous screw fixation or cast immobilization for non-displaced scaphoid fractures. J Bone Joint Surg Am 2001;83:483–8.
15. Brydie A, Raby N. Early MRI in the management of clinical scaphoid fracture. Br J Radiol 2003;76:296–300.
16. Linscheid RL, Weber ER. Scaphoid fractures and nonunion. In: Cooney WP, Linscheid RL, Dobyns JH, editors. The wrist: diagnosis and operative treatment. St Louis (MO): Mosby; 1998. p. 385–430.
17. Gellman H, Caputo R, Carter V, et al. Comparison of short and long thumb-spica casts for non-displaced fractures of the carpal scaphoid. J Bone Joint Surg Am 1989;71(3):354–7.
18. Cooney WP, Dobyns JH, Linscheid RL. Fractures of the scaphoid: a rational approach to management. Clin Orthop 1980;149:90–7.
19. Hung LK, Pang KW. Percutaneous screw fixation of acute scaphoid fractures. J Hand Surg 1994;19(Suppl 1):26.
20. Hung LK. Percutaneous screw fixation of acute scaphoid fractures. HKJOS 1998;2(1):54–7.
21. Hung LK, Pang KW, Ho PC. Anatomical guidelines for safe percutaneous screw fixation of scaphoid fractures. International Proceedings, 6th Congress of IFSSH. Helsinki, Finland; 1995. p. 797–800.
22. Bushnell BD, McWilliams AD, Messer TM. Complications in dorsal percutaneous cannulated screw fixation of non-displaced scaphoid waist fractures. J Hand Surg Am 2007;32(6):827–33.
23. Slade JF III, Taksali S, Safanda J. Combined fractures of the scaphoid and distal radius: a revised treatment rationale using percutaneous and arthroscopic techniques. Hand Clin 2005;21:427–41.
24. Bedi A, Jebson PJL, Hayden RJ, et al. Internal fixation of acute, non-displaced scaphoid waist fractures via a limited dorsal approach: an assessment of radiographic and functional outcomes. J Hand Surg Am 2007;32:326–33.
25. Mack GR, Bosse MJ, Gerberman RH. The natural history of scaphoid nonunion. J Bone Joint Surg Am 1984;66:504–9.
26. Ruby LK, Stinson J, Belsky MR. The natural history of scaphoid nonunion: a review of 55 cases. J Bone Joint Surg Am 1985;67:428–32.
27. Lindstrom G, Nystrom A. Natural history of scaphoid nonunion, with special reference to "asymptomatic" cases. J Hand Surg Br 1992;17:697–700.
28. Cooney WP. Scaphoid fractures: current treatments and techniques. Instr Course Lect 2003;52:197.

29. Herbert TJ, Fisher WE. Management of the fractured scaphoid using a new bone screw. J Bone Joint Surg Br 1984;66:114–23.

30. Filan SL, Herbert TJ. Herbert screw fixation of scaphoid fractures. J Bone Joint Surg Br 1996;78: 519–29.

31. Compson JP, Waterman JK, Spencer JD. Dorsal avulsion fractures of the scaphoid: diagnostic implications and applied anatomy. J Hand Surg Br 1993; 18:58–61.

32. Compson JP. The radiological anatomy of the scaphoid. Part I: osteology. J Hand Surg Br 1994; 22:183–7.

33. Compson JP, Waterman JK, Heatley FW. The radiological anatomy of the scaphoid. Part 2: radiology. J Hand Surg Br 1997;22:8–15.

34. Amadio PC, Berquist TH, Smith DK, et al. Scaphoid malunion. J Hand Surg Am 1989;14:679–87.

35. Ho PC, Hung LK, Lung TK. Acute ligamentous injury in scaphoid fracture. J Bone Joint Surg 2000; 82(Suppl I):82.

36. Garcia-Elias M. Kinetic analysis of carpal stability during grip. Hand Clin 1997;13:151–8.

37. Kobayashi M, Garcia-Elias M, Nagy L. Axial loading induces rotation of proximal carpal row bones around unique screw-displacement axes. J Biomech 1997;30:1165–7.

38. Kobayashi M, Berger RA. Kinematic analysis of scapholunate interosseous ligament repair. Orthop Trans 1995;19:129.

39. Linscheid RL, Dobyn JH, Beabout JW, et al. Traumatic instability of the wrist. Diagnosis, classification, pathomechanics. J Bone Joint Surg Am 1972;54:1612–32.

40. Taleisnik J. Carpal instability. J Bone Joint Surg Am 1988;70:1262–7.

41. Viegas SF, Tencer AF, Cantrell J. Load transfer characteristics of the wrist. II. Perilunate instability. J Hand Surg Am 1987;12:978–85.

42. McCallister WV, Knight J, Kaliappan R, et al. Central placement of the screw in simulated fractures of the scaphoid waist; a biomechanical study. J Bone Joint Surg Am 2003;85:72–7.

43. Dodds SD, Panjabi MM, Slade JF III. Screw fixation of scaphoid fractures: a biomechanical assessment of screw length and screw augmentation. J Hand Surg Am 2006;31:405–13.

44. Goddard NJ. Percutaneous scaphoid fixation: volar traction approach. In: Slusky DJ, Slade JF III, editors. The scaphoid. New York: Thieme; 2011. p. 85–91.

45. Compson JP. Scaphoid fracture patterns and their natural history. In: Guillaume Herzberg, editors. Scaphoïde Carpien 2010. Fractures et Pseudarthroses. Guilaume Herzherg: Sauramps Medical; 61–3 [in French].

The Use of Thermal Shrinkage for Scapholunate Instability

Jonathan R. Danoff, MD[a],*, John W. Karl, MD, MPH[a],
Michael V. Birman, MD[a], Melvin P. Rosenwasser, MD[b]

KEYWORDS

- Radiofrequency shrinkage
- Scapholunate interosseous ligament • Arthroscopy

Scapholunate interosseous ligament (SLIL) instability is the most common form of carpal instability.[1] There is a lack of consensus among hand surgeons as to the appropriate treatment of various stages.[2] Wrist arthroscopy is the gold standard for diagnosis and has allowed for a more nuanced understanding of the continuum of scapholunate (SL) instability.[3] The sensitivity in diagnosis of the spectrum of SLIL injury is possible because of the direct inspection of the ligament from the radiocarpal and midcarpal portals, including palpation and stress testing to assess integrity of the ligament.[4]

A characteristic clinical pattern has been identified that includes chronic dorsal wrist pain especially under loading in wrist extension, a positive Watson test (scaphoid shift test), or apprehension with pain during the examination but without a reduction clunk, and normal static motion studies and grip view radiographs without SL diastasis, and normal magnetic resonance imaging (MRI). This pattern describes a predynamic SL ligament attenuation, which may be either a Geissler grade 1 or 2 lesion (**Table 1**). In Geissler 1 and 2 lesions, there is no to minimal instability because of ligament attenuation without disruption. Grade 3 and 4 lesions represent partial and complete tears with greater degrees of carpal instability. Capsular shrinkage has special application in the treatment of grade 1 and 2 tears.[5] This early but symptomatic ligamentous injury has been successfully treated with arthroscopic thermal collagen shrinkage.[5–8] In this procedure, nonablative thermal energy is discretely and carefully applied to the volar SLIL through midcarpal arthroscopy. The physical heat denaturation of collagen shrinks the ligament.[9] This article reviews the background and results of thermal treatment of predynamic instability of the SLIL. Case examples are discussed as well as a series of patients treated with our protocol for this injury.

ANATOMY OF THE SL COMPLEX

The wrist is a complex structure comprised of intercalated carpal bones stabilized by a web of intrinsic intercarpal ligaments and extrinsic capsular ligaments. The wrist has been described as 2 separate rows, with the proximal row comprised of the scaphoid, lunate, and triquetrum, and the distal

The authors have nothing to disclose with regard to the subject of this manuscript (J.R.D., J.W.K., M.V.B). Melvin P. Rosenwasser, MD serves as a paid consultant for Stryker and Biomet, and has received royalties from Biomet. He serves on the editorial board of the *American Journal of Orthopedics* and serves as a board member for the Foundation for Orthopedic Trauma and Osteosynthesis and Trauma Care Foundation.
[a] Department of Orthopaedic Surgery, Columbia University Medical Center, 622 West 168th Street, PH-1164, New York, NY 10032, USA
[b] Orthopaedic Hand and Trauma Services, Department of Orthopaedic Surgery, Columbia University College of Physicians & Surgeons, 622 West 168th Street, PH-1119, New York, NY 10032, USA
* Corresponding author.
E-mail address: ttc@columbia.edu

Hand Clin 27 (2011) 309–317
doi:10.1016/j.hcl.2011.06.005
0749-0712/11/$ – see front matter © 2011 Elsevier Inc. All rights reserved.

Table 1
Geissler arthroscopic grading system

Grade	Radiocarpal SLIL	Midcarpal Instability
I	Hemorrhage of SLIL, no attenuation	None
II	Incomplete partial or full substance tear, no attenuation	Slight gap (<width of 3-mm probe)
III	Ligament attenuation, incomplete partial or small full substance tear	Probe can be passed between carpal bones
IV	Complete tear	Gross instability, 2.7-mm arthroscope can be passed between SL gap (drive-through sign)

From Geissler WB, Freeland AE, Savoie FH, et al. Intracarpal soft-tissue lesions associated with an intra-articular fracture of the distal end of the radius. J Bone Joint Surg Am 1996;78(3):363; with permission.

row comprised of the trapezium, trapezoid, capitate, and hamate. The scaphoid motion is controlled by numerous intrinsic and extrinsic ligaments, including the SLIL, radioscaphocapitate ligament, scaphotrapeziotrapezoid ligament, scaphocapitate ligament, and dorsal intercarpal ligament.[10] The scaphoid acts as the intercalary link between the carpal rows, to coordinate relative motion between the 2 rows and the bones of the forearm.

The SLIL is a C-shaped structure enveloping the dorsal, proximal, and palmar aspects of the articulation between the scaphoid and the lunate. Berger showed the three-dimensional anatomy of its composite parts (**Fig. 1**).[11] The SL joint and its stability can be assessed arthroscopically from the radiocarpal and midcarpal perspectives, which defines and helps to correlate the clinical and radiographic examinations. The Geissler arthroscopic classification, which includes a visual and tactile provocative examination, has led to a more anatomic understanding of the continuum of SL instability.[5] This classification quantifies the resultant instability and not the size of the tear. The dorsal and palmar portions of the SLIL are true ligamentous structures, whereas the proximal portion (often referred to as the membranous portion) is thin and structurally insignificant and

composed mainly of fibrocartilaginous tissue.[11] Biomechanically, the 3 portions of the SLIL have different material properties, with the dorsal portion of the ligament having the highest load to ultimate failure, followed by the palmar portion, and then the proximal portion.[12]

We have performed a cadaver wrist arthroscopy followed by gross dissection to document the area of the SLIL that is heated with a radiofrequency probe. It is possible to reach the volar SLIL with the probe at the depths of the capsular recess of the SLIL as seen through the midcarpal joint. Thermal shrinkage was specifically performed through the midcarpal portal, targeting both the confluence of the distal radioscaphocapitate ligament and the volar portion of the SLIL. Subsequent dissection of this specimen was performed through a dorsal approach. The proximal carpal row was dissected from the specimen en bloc, maintaining the intrinsic ligaments, and then the capitate was removed. The area that was heated was visible, and we confirmed that the radiofrequency probe placed from a dorsal midcarpal portal was located at the distal radioscaphocapitate ligament and the volar portion of the SLIL, as seen in **Fig. 2**.

DEFINITION AND CLASSIFICATION OF SL INSTABILITY

Cadaveric studies of sequential ligament sectioning have shown that the SLIL is the primary ligament responsible for stabilization of the SL joint.[13–17] Routine radiographs after wrist injury are insufficient to exclude ligament injuries (**Fig. 3**).[18,19] If the clinical examination shows focal dorsal pain at the SL interval, a stress or clenched fist posteroanterior (PA) radiograph should be obtained. If there is no increase in SL diastasis, this has been termed a predynamic instability. The SL ligament complex can be catastrophically disrupted as in a perilunate dislocation or incrementally partially injured, leading to the ultimate and familiar static SL diastasis with or without lunate extension or dorsal intercarpal segmental instability (DISI). Arthrography, even assisted by computer tomography, has largely been supplanted by high-resolution MRI, but often its sensitivity is low for partial ligament injuries or chondral damage. The most sensitive and specific way to assess the degree of SL instability is via wrist arthroscopy (**Fig. 4**).[20]

Three patterns of SL instability are recognized based on symptoms, examination, and imaging. These patterns are predynamic, dynamic, and static, and they reflect the degrees of injury to the SLIL and its secondary stabilizing ligaments. When the ligament is only stretched or partially ruptured,

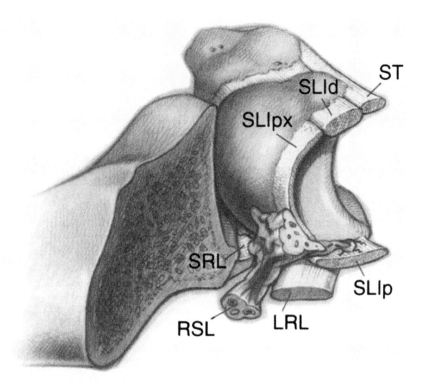

Fig. 1. Anatomy of the SLIL. The scaphoid has been removed to show the 3 main portions of the SLIL. We aim the radiofrequency probe toward the palmar portion of the SLIL (SLIp). (*From* Berger RA. The gross and histologic anatomy of the scapholunate interosseous ligament. J Hand Surg Am 1996;21(2):170–8; with permission.)

Watson termed this predynamic or occult instability. This instability can correspond to a Geissler grade 1 or 2 injury. A patient with predynamic instability has focal pain at the SL joint, usually with normal imaging, including grip stress views. Dynamic radiographic instability is present in patients with normal alignment on unloaded routine radiographs, but an increased SL gap ($\geq$3 mm) with an anteroposterior grip stress view and it is usually consistent with a Geissler grade 3 injury. Often, instability is secondary to incompetence of the secondary stabilizers of the SL joint, including the volar extrinsic (radiolunate, radioscaphocapitate),[18,21] distal intrinsic (scaphotrapezial),[13,22] or dorsal intercarpal ligament. A static SL diastasis or DISI deformity indicates a chronic lesion with attenuation of secondary supporting ligaments, often with extreme lunate extension, and may be associated with some degree of articular degeneration.[23] Static SL instability with a DISI deformity is known to progress to osteoarthritis because of the abnormal loading patterns and mechanics.[24] This pattern of progressive arthritic change has been termed SL advanced collapse (SLAC) arthritis.[25] The acknowledgment of the natural history of SL instability has led to better and more accurate diagnoses via the arthroscope with the goal of earlier treatment and perhaps better outcomes.

HISTORICAL BACKGROUND ON RADIOFREQUENCY SHRINKAGE

Ligaments contain a high concentration of collagen fibers. After thermal-controlled injury, the collagen

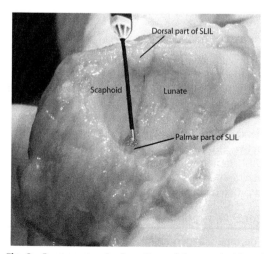

Fig. 2. Gross anatomic dissection of the scaphoid and lunate with radiofrequency probe simulating the portion of the palmar SL ligament and capsular ligament to be thermally shrunk (*dotted area*).

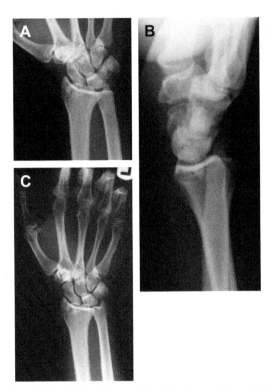

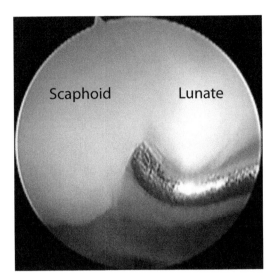

Fig. 4. Intraoperative radiocarpal view of a patient showing the attenuated and partially torn membranous portion of the SL ligament as viewed from the radiocarpal joint.

Fig. 3. (A–C) A 38-year-old patient experienced 8 months of dorsal radial wrist pain after a motor vehicle accident. Symptoms were treated conservatively with splinting and cortisone injections without benefit. New radiographs were obtained. (A) PA image, unstressed with no discernable SL diastasis. (B) Lateral radiograph with normal SL angle indicating no abnormal carpal rotation. (C) Clenched fist PA image showing no change in width of SL interval or SL step-off.

fibers denature and shrink.[6,9] The temperature required to achieve the effect is about 70°C to 80°C and to avoid tissue ablation should not exceed 100°C. Mechanically, this shrinkage tightens (shortens) the supporting ligaments and this affects the relative motion between the scaphoid and lunate when examined clinically and at arthroscopy. In vitro, capsular tissue has been shown to shrink by approximately 9% to 50% depending on the probe and type of tissue. The collagen stiffness is reduced to approximately 20% of normal after shrinkage and returns to normal in about 2 months.[26] This heat injury is delivered by a monopolar or bipolar radiofrequency probe, which delivers nondestructive energy to a discrete area. This technique works best with attenuated ligaments that are in continuity. Tissue repair occurs by vascular invasion and fibroblastic activity. Thermal shrinkage has been used in experimental and clinical settings to alter capsuloligamentous mechanical properties including the joint capsule (glenohumeral, patellofemoral), ligaments (medial collateral ligament of the knee), and tendons (patellar and extensor tendons, Achilles tendon).[27] What has been learned is that discrete or punctate heating promotes better healing after shrinkage by leaving islands of normal tissue and that tissue after shrinking requires immobilization. In the wrist joint, we advocate Kirschner wire (K-wire) pinning to prevent excessive stretching before healing and remodelling. Radiofrequency shrinkage is the treatment of chronic predynamic SL instability and is facilitated by 2-mm probes that are curved at the tip and can navigate around the midcarpal joint.

Indications

Thermal collagen shrinkage is indicated for a patient with graded Geissler grade 1 or 2 instability, who has failed conservative management as defined later. In particular, it may be most useful in partial membranous tears or ligament redundancy. If the surgeon documents excessive motion between the scaphoid and lunate and there is no DISI, radiofrequency thermal collagen shrinkage can tighten the intact portions of the SLIL and improve carpal kinematics.

Contraindications

Thermal collagen shrinkage is contraindicated as an isolated procedure in the presence of static carpal instability, in patients with repairable ligament tears, and in patients with posttraumatic arthritis (advanced SLAC).[28]

MODIFICATION OF THE WATSON SCAPHOID SHIFT TEST

The senior author has used an elaboration and extension of the Watson classic scaphoid shift test in the assessment of patients with predynamic instability. Watson described applying pressure from the palmar side of the volar distal scaphoid pole as the scaphoid is pushed out of its distal radius fossa when the wrist is brought from ulnar into radial deviation.[29] Watson and colleagues[29] designate a positive test when "in patients with ligamentous laxity, the combined stresses of thumb pressure and normal motion of adjacent carpus may be sufficient to force the scaphoid out of the elliptical fossa and up onto the dorsal rim of the radius." Our modification of the classic test uses the same maneuver, but rather than subluxation, the patient experiences reproducible symptoms of pain and apprehension. This clinical finding, not previously described in the literature, is consistent in our experience with predynamic instability, and is later confirmed if subsequent wrist arthroscopy is performed.

NONOPERATIVE TREATMENT

The typical patient presents with focal dorsal wrist pain over the SL joint that corresponds to the 3 to 4 arthroscopic portal. Pain is provoked by firm palpation and by extreme wrist extension under load such as doing a push-up or pushing out of a chair. The Watson scaphoid shift test, discussed in the previous section, is painful and may or may not generate a reduction clunk. As part of our standard workup, we obtain PA and lateral radiographs in neutral rotation, as well as PA grip views (see **Fig. 3**). Stable painful wrists (predynamic instability) are assumed after obtaining normal static and stress radiographs. Unstable wrists with tears shown on grip films or cineradiography only (dynamic instability) have abnormal carpal alignment on stress radiographs (eg, pronated PA grip), but normal alignment on unloaded routine radiographs. Unstable wrists with static instability on routine plain films are obvious and thus not misinterpreted. An MRI scan is often obtained, but should be obtained with a dedicated wrist coil and thin-slice acquisition for best sensitivity. In predynamic SL instability, the SLIL is intact but the MRI may show dorsal synovitis or even a small ganglion.

These patients with predynamic instability are splinted and have activity modification, and they are observed for 6 months or more. Occasionally corticosteroid injections are given, but response is limited. The persistence of pain and functional limitations beyond 6 months in such a patient is our indication for wrist arthroscopy and radiofrequency capsuloligamentous shrinkage at the midcarpal joint, specifically targeting the volar SL ligament.

Arthroscopy is the gold standard for assessment of the spectrum of SL ligament injury. Arthroscopic visualization and palpation of the SLIL and accessory capsular ligaments from the radiocarpal and midcarpal portals defines the injury pattern and severity. The Geissler classification is based on the amount of provocative diastasis judged by utilization of a blunt 2-mm hook. Step-off SL incongruity and slight diastasis (Geissler grade 2) is the typical indication for radiofrequency capsular shrinkage. Synovectomy and debridement are performed first through the radiocarpal and midcarpal portals. Previous reports of radiofrequency shrinkage of the membranous portion notwithstanding, we believe that radiofrequency shrinkage of the more important volar SL ligament through the midcarpal portal is an essential part of this procedure and its successful outcome.[6]

SURGICAL TECHNIQUE

Evaluation of the instability is critical for indication of treatment; therefore, arthroscopy through both radiocarpal and midcarpal portals is required to determine the Geissler grade. If the wrist is stable (Geissler grade 1 or 2 injuries) the tear can be debrided by alternating the arthroscope and working instruments between the 3 to 4 and 4 to 5 radiocarpal portals. The torn portion of the SLIL is debrided to stable margins, with care taken to preserve healthy, intact fibers. This objective is facilitated by using the least aggressive shaver such as a full-radius resector, which does not injure healthy intact tissue. After debridement, it is important to reprobe the midcarpal SL articulation to ensure that stability has not been affected.

After debridement of unstable tissue flaps, a unipolar or bipolar radiofrequency probe (Microblator 30, 1.5 mm, Arthrocare, Sunnyvale, CA, USA or SERFAS, Stryker Endoscopy, San Jose, CA, USA) is inserted in the midcarpal joint. Thermal shrinkage is performed on the palmar midcarpal ligaments (**Fig. 5**) and used in its cauterization setting (not ablative) at the junction of the scaphoid and lunate, which corresponds to the distal edge of the palmar SLIL and the radioscaphocapitate ligament (see **Fig. 2**). The ability to bend the tip of the probe slightly facilitates this approach. The radiofrequency probe is used for punctate energy to be applied to the palmar midcarpal ligaments and capsule in a striping motion (**Fig. 6**). The pulsed nature of this application limits heat buildup, and

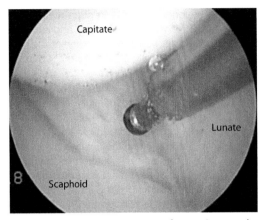

Fig. 5. Midcarpal joint picture of a patient undergoing radiofrequency capsular shrinkage of the palmar midcarpal ligaments.

a pressured irrigation lavage is used to enhance outflow and so facilitate heat dissipation. The radiofrequency shrinkage can be seen to tighten the volar SLIL, which reduces the SL step-off when present and limits or prevents the Geissler probe intrusion between the scaphoid and lunate. Minimal traction required for instrument insertion is to be used to obtain a truer sense of the ligament laxity and its correction. The radiofrequency probe can be used to debride loose fibrillated tissue in its ablative setting as well. After shrinkage, the tightened ligaments have diminished structural properties until healing and it is essential to stabilize the SL and scaphocapitate joints with percutaneous K-wires and immobilization for 4 weeks. At 4 weeks,

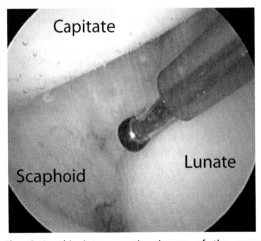

Fig. 6. In this intraoperative image of the same patient seen in **Fig. 3** (before thermal shrinkage), a color change from pearly white to tan/brown is noted after thermal capsular shrinkage of the palmar midcarpal ligaments.

the K-wires are removed and rehabilitation is started, with full activity allowed at 12 weeks.

Other reports of radiofrequency shrinkage in the wrist describe thermal stabilization using monopolar cautery (Oratec, Mountain View, CA, USA) placed through the 4 to 5 radiocarpal portal.[7] This strategy addresses the less important membranous portion of the SL complex. Another study uses a 2.3-mm bipolar probe (Vapr; Mitek, Westwood, MA, USA) again, placed through the 4 to 5 portal.[6] Again, the radiocarpal approach limits access to the volar SLIL. It cannot be seen from this view. We believe it is necessary to approach and instrument the volar SLIL through the midcarpal joint and that concomitant debridement of the membranous portion helps only by relieving the mechanical impingement and resultant synovitis. This cadaver photograph (see **Fig. 2**) shows the volar SLIL, which is visible and shrinkable through the midcarpal access.

PATIENT CASE EXAMPLE

A 33-year-old, right-hand-dominant athlete and high-school football coach injured his right wrist in a fall playing basketball 16 years previously. He reported episodic, severe pain, exacerbated by full wrist extension that limited function. He had a sensation of mechanical instability with clicking and popping, which resulted in swelling. The Watson scaphoid shift test caused apprehension and pain. He had been managed with splints and rest for 16 years. Many activities increased his symptoms such as golf or throwing a football. After an errant divot in golf, he had severe wrist pain. Radiographs were negative and an MRI scan showed a tear of the membranous portion of the SLIL and synovitis. He met the criteria for surgical intervention with arthroscopy and radiofrequency shrinkage. Radiocarpal inspection confirmed a membranous tear of the SL ligament. Midcarpal viewing showed hypermobility of the SL joint, which was graded Geissler 2. Radiofrequency thermal shrinkage was performed to the volar SLIL. Transarticular SL and scaphocapitate K-wires stabilized the repair.

At 3 months, his wrist was stable with a negative Watson test and he subjectively felt that the wrist was "tighter." At 4 months, he had no pain and equivalent strength to the contralateral wrist and had returned to all his vocational and avocational activities without restriction. These activities included throwing footballs as a high-school coach and weight lifting, which was impossible before surgery. At 12 months, he had a DASH (Disabilities of the Arm, Shoulder, and Hand) score

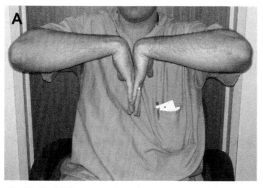
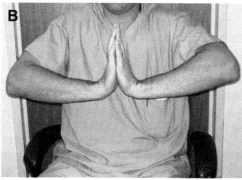

Fig. 7. Clinical follow-up of patient case example 12 months after arthroscopic debridement, thermal shrinkage, and temporary K-wire fixation. Patient maintains 83% wrist flexion (*A*) and 93% wrist extension (*B*) compared with normal contralateral side.

of 2.5, wrist extension of 70°, flexion of 75°, and pronation and supination to 90° (**Fig. 7**).

RESULTS AND COMPLICATIONS

Darlis and colleagues[6] examined 16 patients (mean age, 34 years) with subacute Geissler grade 1 or 2 SLIL injuries treated by capsular shrinkage and only 2 weeks of immobilization. At 19 months, there were 14 excellent/good results and 2 fair/poor results using the modified Mayo wrist score.[6] Hirsh

and colleagues[7] treated 10 patients (mean age, 37 years) with Geissler grade 2 SLIL injuries using capsular shrinkage and 4 to 6 weeks of immobilization. Symptom duration was greater than 6 months in 8 patients. At 28 months the pain had resolved in 9 of 10 patients. Similarly, Shih and Lee[8] studied 19 patients (mean age, 23 years) with chronic symptomatic SL instability. At 28 months after thermal shrinkage, 15 of 19 patients were fully satisfied with the results and returned to their preinjury activity. Four patients had recurrent laxity of the

Table 2
Comparison of our results with published data

	Hirsh and Colleagues[7]	Darlis and Colleagues[6]	Our (Unpublished) Case Series
Number of patients	10	16	8
Average age (y)	37	34	38
Average length of symptoms (mo)	2 (<6)	5	25
Clinical instability	10	13	4
Radiographic instability			
Predynamic	8	16	5
Dynamic	2	0	3
Geissler grade			
1	0	2	1
2	10	14	7
Procedure (postoperative immobilization)	Monopolar thermal shrinkage (4–6 wk)	Debridement + bipolar thermal shrinkage (2 wk)	4 debridement + shrinkage (none) 3 debridement + shrinkage + pinning (6–8 wk)
Average follow-up (mo)	28	19	4–8
Outcome	9/10 pain resolved average DASH score = 20	14 substantial pain relief, 8 pain free, grip 78%, flex/ext 142°	6 good pain relief and minimal loss of motion, 1 wrist fusion

SL joint, which was treated with a dorsal capsulodesis. The loss of wrist motion averaged 5°.

We retrospectively reviewed 8 consecutive cases of SL injury treated with arthroscopic debridement and radiofrequency shrinkage. The patient population averaged 38 years, with symptoms for an average of 25 months before surgery. Four patients had a positive Watson scaphoid shift test. Five patients were predynamic and 3 had dynamic instability. At arthroscopy, 7 were graded Geissler 2 and 1 Geissler 1. Surgery was performed as previously described. Follow-up ranged from 3 to 8 months, with 7 patients reporting reduced pain with preservation of wrist mobility. One patient failed and eventually had a wrist fusion. Our results compare favorably with previous reports (**Table 2**) for thermal collagen shrinkage.[6,7] These preliminary findings suggest that arthroscopic debridement and radiofrequency thermal collagen shrinkage can be an effective treatment of patients with symptomatic predynamic and dynamic SLIL injuries.

SUMMARY

Delayed or missed diagnosis of SLIL instability can lead to persistent symptoms and progressive carpal instability. SLIL injury is a continuum and despite the absence of radiographic or MRI findings can be painful and disabling. Predynamic or dynamic SLIL instability and Geissler grade 1 or 2 SL laxity can be successfully treated with radiofrequency capsuloligamentous shrinkage of the volar SLIL. We recommend transcarpal K-wire fixation of the SL and scaphocapitate joints for 4 weeks to protect the heated ligaments during healing and remodeling. In the case of a patient with predynamic or dynamic instability with a Geissler grade 1 or 2 tear of the SLIL, radiofrequency thermal collagen shrinkage of the volar SLIL and surrounding capsular ligaments is an excellent treatment option. It can be performed with arthroscopic debridement alone or in combination with temporary transarticular pinning, with good to excellent results, as seen in the small case series.

REFERENCES

1. Walsh JJ, Berger RA, Cooney WP. Current status of scapholunate interosseous ligament injuries. J Am Acad Orthop Surg 2002;10(1):32–42.
2. Ruch DS, Poehling GG. Arthroscopic management of partial scapholunate and lunotriquetral injuries of the wrist. J Hand Surg Am 1996;21(3):412–7.
3. Rettig ME, Amadio PC. Wrist arthroscopy. Indications and clinical applications. J Hand Surg Br 1994;19(6):774–7.
4. Dautel G, Goudot B, Merle M. Arthroscopic diagnosis of scapho-lunate instability in the absence of X-ray abnormalities. J Hand Surg Br 1993;18(2):213–8.
5. Geissler WB, Freeland AE, Savoie FH, et al. Intracarpal soft-tissue lesions associated with an intra-articular fracture of the distal end of the radius. J Bone Joint Surg Am 1996;78(3):357–65.
6. Darlis NA, Weiser RW, Sotereanos DG. Partial scapholunate ligament injuries treated with arthroscopic debridement and thermal shrinkage. J Hand Surg Am 2005;30(5):908–14.
7. Hirsh L, Sodha S, Bozentka D, et al. Arthroscopic electrothermal collagen shrinkage for symptomatic laxity of the scapholunate interosseous ligament. J Hand Surg Br 2005;30(6):643–7.
8. Shih JT, Lee HM. Monopolar radiofrequency electrothermal shrinkage of the scapholunate ligament. Arthroscopy 2006;22(5):553–7.
9. Andary J, Arnoczky S. Thermal modification of connective tissue: basic science considerations. In: DeLee JC, Drez D, editors. DeLee and Drez's orthopaedic sports medicine. 2nd edition. Philadelphia: Saunders; 2003. p. 213–24.
10. Berger RA. The anatomy of the ligaments of the wrist and distal radioulnar joints. Clin Orthop Relat Res 2001;(383):32–40.
11. Berger RA. The gross and histologic anatomy of the scapholunate interosseous ligament. J Hand Surg Am 1996;21(2):170–8.
12. Berger RA, Imeada T, Berglund L, et al. Constraint and material properties of the subregions of the scapholunate interosseous ligament. J Hand Surg Am 1999;24(5):953–62.
13. Short WH, Werner FW, Green JK, et al. The effect of sectioning the dorsal radiocarpal ligament and insertion of a pressure sensor into the radiocarpal joint on scaphoid and lunate kinematics. J Hand Surg Am 2002;27(1):68–76.
14. Burgess RC. The effect of rotatory subluxation of the scaphoid on radio-scaphoid contact. J Hand Surg Am 1987;12(5 Pt 1):771–4.
15. Ruch DS, Smith BP. Arthroscopic and open management of dynamic scaphoid instability. Orthop Clin North Am 2001;32(2):233–40, vii.
16. Meade TD, Schneider LH, Cherry K. Radiographic analysis of selective ligament sectioning at the carpal scaphoid: a cadaver study. J Hand Surg Am 1990;15(6):855–62.
17. Blevens AD, Light TR, Jablonsky WS, et al. Radiocarpal articular contact characteristics with scaphoid instability. J Hand Surg Am 1989;14(5):781–90.
18. Short WH, Werner FW, Green JK, et al. Biomechanical evaluation of ligamentous stabilizers of the scaphoid and lunate. J Hand Surg Am 2002;27(6):991–1002.
19. Berger RA, Blair WF, Crowninshield RD, et al. The scapholunate ligament. J Hand Surg Am 1982; 7(1):87–91.

20. Mitsuyasu H, Patterson RM, Shah MA, et al. The role of the dorsal intercarpal ligament in dynamic and static scapholunate instability. J Hand Surg Am 2004; 29(2):279–88.

21. Ruby LK, An KN, Linscheid RL, et al. The effect of scapholunate ligament section on scapholunate motion. J Hand Surg Am 1987;12(5 Pt 1):767–71.

22. Boabighi A, Kuhlmann JN, Kenesi C. The distal ligamentous complex of the scaphoid and the scapholunate ligament. An anatomic, histological and biomechanical study. J Hand Surg Br 1993;18(1):65–9.

23. Watson H, Ottoni L, Pitts EC, et al. Rotary subluxation of the scaphoid: a spectrum of instability. J Hand Surg Br 1993;18(1):62–4.

24. Watson HK, Ryu J. Evolution of arthritis of the wrist. Clin Orthop Relat Res 1986;(202):57–67.

25. Watson HK, Ballet FL. The SLAC wrist: scapholunate advanced collapse pattern of degenerative arthritis. J Hand Surg Am 1984;9(3):358–65.

26. Medvecky MJ, Ong BC, Rokito AS, et al. Thermal capsular shrinkage: basic science and clinical applications. Arthroscopy 2001;17(6):624–35.

27. Dugas JR, Andrews JR. Thermal capsular shrinkage in the throwing athlete. Clin Sports Med 2002;21(4): 771–6.

28. Rosenwasser MP, Riansuwan K. Arthroscopic treatment of scapholunate ligament tears. In: Slutsky DJ, Nagle DJ, editors. Techniques in hand and wrist arthroscopy. Philadelphia: Elsevier; 2007. p. 66–78.

29. Watson HK, Ashmead D 4th, Makhlouf MV. Examination of the scaphoid. J Hand Surg Am 1988;13(5): 657–60.

Arthroscopic Treatment of Scaphotrapeziotrapezoid Osteoarthritis

C. Mathoulin, MD[a],*, F. Darin, MD[b]

KEYWORDS

- STT arthritis • Distal scaphoid resection • Wrist prosthesis

Scaphotrapeziotrapezoid (STT) joint osteoarthritis is less known than other types of wrist arthritis. This disease accounts for only 13% of all wrist arthritis sites.[1] Isolated lesions of this joint are rare and their therapeutic management is hard. The only treatment proposed for long was STT arthrodesis, a procedure of which the technical difficulty has caused numerous complications.[2] Pseudoarthrosis is common, and STT arthrodesis has been incriminated in the occurrence of radioscaphoid osteoarthritis. Techniques of distal resection combined with interposition of biologic tissues such as tendons (flexor carpi radialis) have been described in the 1990s.[3] In other reports, interposition of a palmar or dorsal capsular prosthesis was combined with resection.[4] It was reasonable to carry out such procedures with arthroscopic aid to prevent extensive scar and the instability due to ligament lesions.[5–8]

METHODS

The anatomy of the STT joint is simple. The concavity of the proximal trapeziotrapezoid joint matches the convexity of the scaphoid distal pole. The stabilization of this joint depends on the scaphotrapezial ligament, which is thicker on its palmar face. There are 2 important entities involved in such stabilization: the dorsal capsular reinforcement of the STT ligament and the palmar radioscaphocapitate ligament. This joint has close relationships with the radial artery that comes ahead of the joint and with the dorsal branch of this artery, which crosses back the scaphotrapezoid joint. The terminal branches of the radial nerve also pass in this area.

THE SURGICAL TECHNIQUE

Patients are placed in the supine position. Traction is applied following the thumb axis using a Chinese fingertrap. Traction of 2 to 3 kg is sufficient. The joint is filled first with water via a midcarpal portal. The radial midcarpal portal is selected on principle. This portal allows initiating both the arthroscope and the arthroscopic aid and the examination of the joint (**Fig. 1**). Then the 1–2 midcarpal or STT portal is marked out using a needle. Much attention must be paid to the position of the radial artery and the radial nerve branches. As in any arthroscopic portal realization, small transverse incisions are performed in the skin only; then the joint is reached using a foam rubber forceps so as to prevent any lesion of the important parts in the area. A Spanish working group has described a palmar portal for which we have no experience.[9] Performing direct dorsal portal may be considered, provided the trapezial axis, and the specific round shape of this joint is taken into account. A sucking mechanical drill is inserted via the 1–2 portal. Resection is made, beginning at the internal dorsal side and pursued progressively under visual control until the palmar part of the scaphoid distal tubercle (**Fig. 2**). A resection of at least 2 to 3 mm is necessary. In case no implant has to be inserted, portals are left open or closed simply by Steristrips (3M Health Care, St Paul, MN, USA). In case of pyrocarbon implant interposition, the STT portal is slightly enlarged so as to ease the implant passage. There are 2 implant sizes (small and large; **Fig. 3**). Testing implants are inserted under arthroscopic control. Once the final implant is placed, a knot is performed on the joint capsule and the skin is closed

a Institut de la Main, Clinique Jouvenet, 6 Square Jouvenet, 75016 Paris, France
b Istituto Codivilla Putti, Orthopedica, Via Codivilla 1, 32043 Cortina d'Ampezzo, Italie
* Corresponding author.
E-mail address: cmathoulin@orange.fr

Hand Clin 27 (2011) 319–322
doi:10.1016/j.hcl.2011.05.001

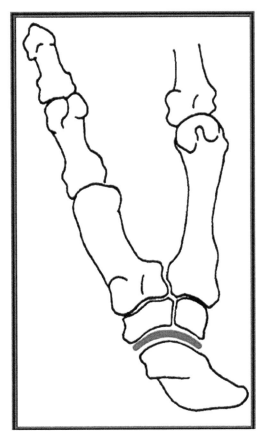

Fig. 1. Outlined particular shape of the STT joint; this shape is to be taken into account when initiating the arthroscope and performing the scaphoid distal resection.

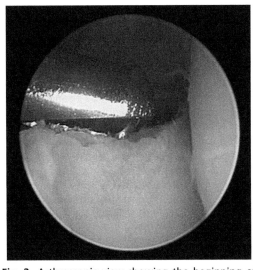

Fig. 2. Arthroscopic view showing the beginning of the resection; the capitatum is on the left, and the distal pole of the scaphoid is at the bottom of the figure.

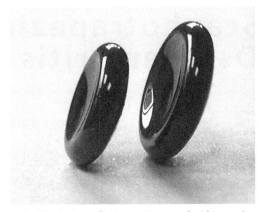

Fig. 3. The 2 sizes of interposition scaphoid trapezium pyrocarbon implants. Notice the concavity of the proximal face that adequately matches the convexity of the scaphoid distal pole.

by separate stitches. Commissural immobilization splint is always fitted for a 3-week period; then, patients can use their hands normally. Most often, rehabilitation is not necessary. From 2002 to 2005, we operated on 26 patients with isolated STT osteoarthritis. All had already undergone unsuccessful preoperative medical treatment combining orthesis-based immobilization, nonsteroidal antiinflammatory therapy, and corticoid infiltration. Treatment duration averaged 8 months (range, 3–18 months). In all patients, radiological assessment showed complete disappearance of the STT joint space. Sometimes, osseous cystic reaction was observed at the level of the scaphoid distal pole. Systematic front and side radiographies were performed so as to measure scapholunate angles and verify that no disaxation was present as a result of a lesion of intrinsic ligaments, which could constitute a reason for absolute contraindication.[10] The trapeziometacarpal joint was of course screened for any arthritic lesion that could also constitute a contraindication.

All patients were reassessed regularly, with an evaluation of mobility, muscle strength, pinch, pain, and return to prior activity. Outcome satisfaction was also assessed.

Data were analyzed in terms of the Green-O'Brien score.[9] When possible, comparisons with the contralateral side were performed.

RESULTS
Isolated Resection of the Scaphoid Distal Pole

The study population includes 13 women with an average age of 58 years (range, 52–64 years). In terms of the Green-O'Brien score, the analysis shows a mean preoperative value of 50, increased to 90 postoperatively (**Table 1**). Only 1 complication

Table 1
According to modified mayo wrist score series results

	Preoperative Value	Postoperative Value
Pain	15	25
Function	15	25
Range of motion	15	25
Grip strength	5	15
Total score	50	90

occurred: a transient dysesthesia on the dorsal side of the thumb because of the irritation of a sensitive radial nerve branch. These dysesthesias resolved spontaneously. We observed a progressive compression of the scaphotrapezial space, but no pain phenomena occurred subsequently. Longer follow-up is necessary to confirm absence of pain recurrence (**Fig. 4**).

Interposition Scaphoid Trapezium Pyrocarbon Implants

We operated on 13 patients using this technique, 12 women and 1 man. Their ages averaged 62 years (range, 48–79 years). All patients presented with disabling pains that worsened for several months and was refractory to conventional therapy, with a significant reduction of muscular and pinch strength and preservation of mobility. The average duration of the follow-up was 20 months (range 11–27 months). Overall mobility was improved in all patients; pain disappeared completely in 12 cases and diminished in 1 case. Two implant dislocations occurred in relation with a therapeutic mistake. In fact, the resection of the distal pole was insufficient, and it left a medial bone wall responsible for inadequate insertion of the implant. Affected patients underwent reintervention by the same technique, including resection and reinsertion of the implant. Patients experienced no other problem postoperatively. No infectious complication had to be reported, and painful phenomena disappeared completely. Muscular strength, that is, grip and pinch, increased in all patients (**Fig. 5**).

DISCUSSION

The outcome quality of such isolated resections is consistent with other results reported in the literature.[6,11] Nevertheless, it seems that progressive compression develops in the axis with time, with an impingement phenomenon at the level of the STT joint.

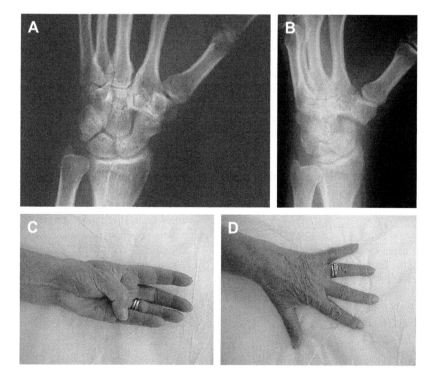

Fig. 4. (*A*) Isolated lesion of the STT joint in a 53-year-old female patient. (*B*) Outcome 4 years after isolated resection. (*C*, *D*) Good overall mobility, and no pain.

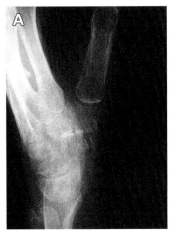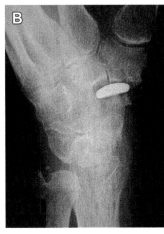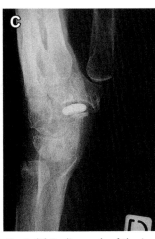

Fig. 5. (*A*) Isolated osteoarthritis of the STT joint in a 61-year-old female patient. (*B*) Radiograph of the inserted implant at 2 weeks. (*C*) Radiograph of the inserted implant at 4 years; the patient uses her hand normally and without experiencing any pain; the implant is still perfectly in place and very stable.

Inserting an interposition scaphoid trapezium pyrocarbon implant is likely to prevent this problem. However, this insertion necessitates strictly conforming to the surgical technique and procedure, in particular, regarding the resection of the distal pole. The advisability of a trapezial and trapezoid proximal resection may be considered because it seems to be more logical, but, from a technical point of view, the proximal part of the trapezium and the trapezoid being much more compact, its resection using miniaturized drills is obviously more difficult. In our 2 series, radiocarpal angles were not modified even at late assessments, after 4 years of follow-up. In case of peritrapezial osteoarthritis, these techniques may not be realized, and concerned patients should undergo preferably combined trapeziectomy and ligamentoplasty.

When the rules of interposition implant insertion are strictly and adequately respected, in particular, when the scaphoid distal pole is sufficiently resected, the outcome quality optimized by the mini-invasive portal access and the arthroscopic assistance suggest selecting some indications, although these should remain rare.

REFERENCES

1. Zemel NP. Traitement de l'arthrose isole de l'articulation scapho-trapézo-trapézoïdienne. In: Saffar PH, editor. La rhizarthrose (monographies du GEM). Paris: Expansion Scientifique Française; 1990. p. 194–202.
2. Frykman EB, Afekenstam F, Wadin K. Triscaphoid arthrodesis and its complications. J Hand Surg Am 1988;13(6):844–9.
3. Linscheid RL, Lirette R, Dobyns JH. L'arthrose dégénérative scapho-trapézienne. In: Saffar PH, editor. La rhizarthrose (monographies du GEM). Paris: Expansion Scientifique Française; 1990. p. 185–94.
4. Garcia-Elias M, Lluch AL, Farreres A. Treatment of scaphotrapeziotrapezoid arthrosis by distal scaphoid resection and capsular interposition arthroplasty. In: Saffar PH, Amadio PC, Foucher G, editors. Current practice in hand surgery. (UK): Martin Dunitz LTD; 1997. p. 181–5.
5. Ashwood N, Bain GI, Fogg Q. Result of arthroscopic debridement for isolated scaphotrapeziotrapezoid arthritis. J Hand Surg Am 2003;28(5):729–32.
6. Moritomo H, Viegas SF, Nakamura K, et al. The scaphotrapezio-trapezoidal joint. J Hand Surg Am 2000;25(5). Part 1: 899–910, Part 2: 911–20.
7. Sonenblum SE, Crisco JJ, Kang L, et al. In vivo motion of the scaphotrapezio-trapezoidal (STT) joint. J Biomech 2004;37(5):645–52.
8. Drewniany J, Palmer AK. Le complexe ligamentaire scapho-trapézien et l'arthrose de l'articulation scapho-trapézo-trapézoïdienne. In: Saffar PH, editor. La rhizarthrose (monographies du GEM). Paris: Expansion Scientifique Française; 1990. p. 18–24.
9. Perez Carro L, Golanó P. The radial portal for scaphotrapeziotrapezoid arthroscopy. Arthroscopy 2003;19:547–53.
10. Brown Crosby E, Linscheid RL, Dobyns JH. Scaphotrapezial trapezoidal arthrosis. J Hand Surg Am 1978;3(3):223–34.
11. Green DP, O'Brien ET. Open reduction of carpal dislocations: indications and operative techniques. J Hand Surg 1978;3:250–65.

Arthroscopic Assessment of Avascular Necrosis

Gregory I. Bain, MBBS, FRACS, PhD[a,b,c],*,
Adam W. Durrant, MBChB, FRACS[a]

KEYWORDS

- Kienbock disease • Arthroscopy • Lunate
- Avascular necrosis

Avascular necrosis of the lunate is attributed to Robert Kienbock, who first described lunatomalacia in 1910.[1] At the time of preparing this article, it is the 100-year anniversary of his description. The cause of avascular necrosis of the lunate is uncertain, but a common theory persists that it is caused by disruption of the vascular supply to the lunate. The cause of this disruption is the source of considerable debate. Kienbock initially felt that the collapse of the lunate, which he noted on radiograph, was caused by repetitive trauma to the lunate from work-related activities. This opinion was backed up by the work of Muller in 1920 who coined the term occupational lunatomalacia. Muller was also the first to notice the association with an ulnar minus variance and this was subsequently supported by the work of Hulten in 1928.[1,2] Mirabello and colleagues[3] believed that a flat distal radius (with less than the normal 23 degrees of radial inclination) may also be a factor, increasing loading on the lunate. Various other investigators have studied features pertaining to the lunate that may predispose to avascular necrosis, such as trabecular pattern, number of facets, and angle in relation to the distal radius.[1,3]

Kienbock disease is more common in men, and typically presents between the ages of 20 and 40 years. Patients present with wrist swelling, pain, and restricted range of motion. These symptoms, in turn, lead to difficulty with activities of daily living.

Initial diagnosis can be difficult because the findings may be subtle and plain film radiographs are often normal in the early stages of the condition. With the increased availability of magnetic resonance imaging (MRI), early diagnosis has been facilitated. MRI is capable of detecting the subtle early changes in Kienbock disease, such as edema and decreased blood flow (ischemia). Initially, the lunate has an increased signal secondary to edema; this changes to an almost total lack of signal as the bone becomes ischemic and then necrotic (**Fig. 1**). With MRI, it is also possible to detect the sagittal fracture lines that may complicate avascular necrosis of the lunate.

Computed tomography (CT) scans have also been used to assess the lunate in Kienbock disease (**Fig. 2**). The advantages of CT are its low cost and better assessment of the joint surfaces and osseous involvement of the lunate. It is also useful for assessing fractures of the lunate.[4]

Avascular necrosis of the lunate is a process that is not well understood. Most of the investigation into avascular necrosis of bone has been performed on the femoral head, and the findings have been extrapolated to various other bones such as the lunate. However, the various bones that are susceptible to avascular necrosis often have dissimilar functions, and extrapolation of findings in the femoral head may lead to false conclusions about the cause of avascular necrosis of the

Support from industry and pharmaceutical sources; nil.
The authors have nothing to disclose.
[a] Modbury Hospital, Smart Road, Modbury, SA 5092, Australia
[b] Department of Orthopaedic Surgery, University of Adelaide, North Terrace, SA 5000, Australia
[c] Royal Adelaide Hospital, North Terrace, SA 5000, Australia
* Corresponding author. 196 Melbourne Street, North Adelaide, SA 5006, Australia.
E-mail address: greg@gregbain.com.au

Hand Clin 27 (2011) 323–329
doi:10.1016/j.hcl.2011.05.006
0749-0712/11/$ – see front matter © 2011 Elsevier Inc. All rights reserved.

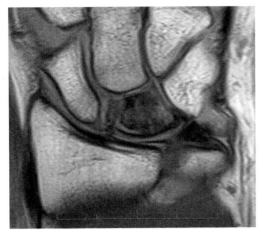

Fig. 1. MRI scan showing the lunate with some fragmentation, a subchondral fracture extending distally. The articular cartilage is partly irregular. At this stage, the resolution of the articular cartilage is not sufficient to recommend treatment.

lunate, and from there may lead to flawed management strategies. Theories as to the cause of avascular necrosis can usually be classified into 3 groups, again as extrapolated from the causes of avascular necrosis in the femoral head. Death of bone can be attributed to a lack of a blood supply either caused by arterial occlusion, or a decrease in venous outflow leading to secondary venous congestion. Some investigators have suggested that raised intraosseous pressure could be a third cause of avascular necrosis. A fourth

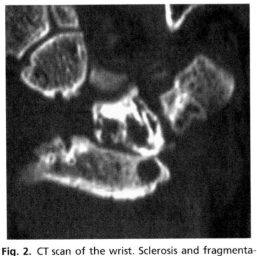

Fig. 2. CT scan of the wrist. Sclerosis and fragmentation of the lunate. Full-thickness loss of the articular cartilage of the lunate and lunate facet must exist for there to be bone-on-bone degenerative arthritis with complete loss of the joint space.

theory has been postulated for the lunate: repetitive microtrauma secondary to repeated abnormal loading of the bone.

After the initial insult has ceased or been rectified, the bone undergoes a process of revascularization through angiogenesis. This process takes a considerable period of time and hence there is resorption of dead bone ahead of the advancing angiogenesis. At this point, the survival of the articular surface depends on the ability of the affected bone to lay down new subchondral bone to support the overlying articular cartilage before collapse and fracturing of the joint surface can occur. The articular cartilage is usually unaffected because it is mainly nourished by the synovial fluid and hence, in the hip, strategies to decrease load on the affected femoral head have been used. This information has been extrapolated to the lunate and early management of avascular necrosis of the lunate is often with rest and splintage. Articular collapse is an irreversible process that leads to secondary degenerative changes in the joint.

Avascular necrosis of the femoral head is often classified using the system as set out by Ficat.[5] This classification has undergone many modifications, especially with the advent of MRI. Because of a lack of dedicated classification systems, that of Ficat[5] is often extrapolated to different bones because of a lack of a specific classification system for that area.[5]

Traditionally, Kienbock disease has been classified according to the system set out by Lichtman. It relies on assessment of plain radiographs of the wrist to reveal the degree of lunate collapse and its rotational alignment in relation to the adjacent scaphoid. The reliability of this system has been questioned, but there are few alternative classification systems available to clinicians.[6,7] Classification using radiographs has also been questioned regarding its usefulness to the clinician in deciding on an appropriate management strategy. It has also been modified several times to include extra stages to include the use of MRI imaging.

The use of wrist arthroscopy for the treatment of Kienbock disease was first described by Menth-Chiari and colleagues[8] in 1999. Their model was to use arthroscopy to assess the articular surfaces and also to debride the necrotic lunate and perform a limited synovectomy. In their study, all patients were either Lichtman grade IIIA or IIIB, and all experienced relief of their painful mechanical symptoms. Bain and Begg,[9] in 2006, furthered this work by introducing an arthroscopic grading system for Kienbock disease. Bain and Begg's[9] classification system uses arthroscopy to grade the degenerative changes in the radiolunate and lunocapitate joints (**Table 1**). They then made recommendations for treatment depending on the changes on each articular surface. The advantage of this system is that it is a direct visual assessment of the articulations of the lunate, and, with the use of a probe, the degree of softening of the articular surface can also be assessed. Correlating this arthroscopic assessment with the traditional investigations can help the clinician make better-informed management decisions.

Arthroscopic assessment is performed using standard wrist arthroscopic techniques.[10] The operative limb is suspended in finger traps. A high arm tourniquet is used. Traction (5 kg) is used to provide joint distraction and is applied via a padded sling passed over the tourniquet with the weight suspended on a hook. Standard 3-4, 6R, and midcarpal portals are used. A general assessment of the radiocarpal and midcarpal joints is performed. The presence or absence of synovitis or loose bodies is noted. The radiocarpal and capitolunate surfaces of the lunate are assessed, as are the corresponding articular facets on the distal radius and the head of the capitate. The surfaces are palpated with a probe and the presence of softening, a floating (unsupported) articular surface, or gross degenerative changes are noted. Any associated fractures of the lunate can also be assessed.[9] At the same time, debridement of the joints can be performed if no further surgical intervention is planned.

Bain and Begg's[9] classification is based on the number of nonfunctional articular surfaces. The investigators define the normal arthroscopic appearance of the cartilage as having a white, smooth, glistening appearance. Minor fibrillation is still classified as a normal articular surface. The subchondral bone must be firm to palpation, with no signs of softening. Articular surfaces that display extensive fibrillation, fissuring, localized or extensive articular loss, a floating articular surface, or fracture should be considered abnormal. The degree of synovitis is not considered in this arthroscopic classification system, but it usually correlates with the degree of articular damage. It has been noted that the degenerative changes in the lunate usually develop on the convex, proximal, surface of the lunate first. As these changes become more pronounced, the lunate facet of the radius becomes affected.

It has been observed by the authors that plain film radiographs often underestimate the severity of the changes in avascular necrosis of the lunate, and that the arthroscopic findings often change the recommendation of treatment. MRI is useful for assessing the stage of avascular necrosis and detecting fracturing of the lunate, but it is not sensitive enough to accurately assess the articular surfaces. The advantage of direct arthroscopic assessment is that it allows the surgeon to visually inspect and palpate the articular surfaces.

Table 1
Bain and Begg arthroscopic classification of avascular necrosis of the lunate

Grade	Description	Recommended Treatment
Grade 0	All articular surfaces are functional	Synovectomy Joint leveling Vascularized bone graft Forage
Grade 1	One nonfunctional surface Usually the proximal lunate	Radioscapholunate fusion Proximal row carpectomy
Grade 2a	Two nonfunctional surfaces. Proximal lunate and lunate facet of radius	Radioscapholunate fusion
Grade 2b	Two nonfunctional surfaces. Proximal and distal surfaces of the lunate	Proximal row carpectomy Lunate replacement
Grade 3	Three nonfunctional surfaces. Likely to be the proximal and distal surfaces of the lunate and the lunate facet of the radius with a preserved capitate articular surface	Hemiarthroplasty or Total wrist fusion or Wrist replacement
Grade 4	Four nonfunctional articular surfaces	Total wrist fusion Wrist replacement

Synovectomy is performed in all patients at time of arthroscopy.
From Bain GI, Begg M. Arthroscopic assessment and classification of Kienbock's disease. Tech Hand Up Extrem Surg 2006;10(1):11; with permission.

Traditionally, the first line of treatment has been nonoperative, with the use of corticosteroid injections, wrist splints, oral analgesics, and activity modification. Nonoperative treatment is still popular in some centers but is losing favor because these therapies do not reverse the progression of lunate collapse. Surgical interventions have focused on unloading the lunate to try to prevent collapse. Traditional procedures include radial shortening, ulnar lengthening, capitate shortening, and scaphotrapeziotrapezoid (STT) or scaphocapitate joint arthrodesis.[3,11] Replacement arthroplasty has been attempted using a variety of materials including silicone, titanium, and methylmethacrylate cement.[12] Various revascularization procedures have been attempted using donor vessels and bone blocks from the distal radius and metacarpals. Limited wrist fusions in the form of radioscapholunate arthrodesis have also been attempted. Core decompression has also been attempted to address the raised intraosseous pressure and to encourage angiogenesis.[13] This can now be performed as an arthroscopic-assisted procedure.

ARTICULAR APPROACH TO TREATMENT

Traditionally, Kienbock disease has been managed based on the radiological osseous findings as defined by Lichtman's classification.[2] The authors have used an articular-based approach to determine surgical treatment (**Fig. 3**, see **Table 1**). Functional and nonfunctional articular surfaces are identified and the Bain and Begg classification determined. The aim of the surgical treatment is to leave the carpus articulating with functional articular surfaces, while maintaining a functional range of motion. Arthroscopy is a grading tool and can also be a therapeutic tool. At arthroscopy, synovectomy and/or debridement can be performed. However, the authors proceed directly to a reconstructive procedure to remove or fuse nonfunctional articulations if identified.

THE ARTHROSCOPIC GRADING SYSTEM

The specific components of the arthroscopic grading system are as follows (**Fig. 4**).

Grade 0

All articular surfaces are functional.

An arthroscopic synovectomy is performed, because the surgeon is perfectly positioned to do so. An extra-articular unloading procedure may be indicated. If there is negative ulnar variance, then a radial shortening osteotomy is performed. For neutral or positive ulnar variance,

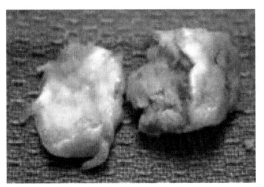

Fig. 3. Excised lunate, with thin and ulcerated articular cartilage from a patient with a grade 2B lunate. Note the necrotic bone and thinned ulcerated nonfunctional articular cartilage. Previously a surgeon would manage this patient based on the radiological osseous findings. It is the authors' view that the nonfunctional articular cartilage, if left in-situ, will lead to a poor prognosis and that the necrotic bone, which is communicating with the joint, will elute necrotic chemical factors, together leading to a compromised outcome.

a capitate shortening procedure can be performed. A revascularization procedure could also be indicated in this group. The authors have also managed 2 patients with a forage operation. This operation involved arthroscopic-assisted drilling of the lunate.[13] The 2 patients have had a satisfactory outcome when reviewed at 6 years' follow-up.

Grade 1

Nonfunctional proximal lunate articular surface only.

Proximal row carpectomy or radioscapholunate fusion may be indicated.

Grade 2

Two nonfunctional articular surfaces.

Grade 2A
The proximal articular surface of the lunate and the lunate fossa are both nonfunctional. A radioscapholunate fusion will remove both nonfunctional articular surfaces and enable the wrist to articulate through the normal midcarpal joint.

Grade 2B
The proximal and distal articular surfaces of the lunate are nonfunctional. This condition typically occurs when there is a coronal fracture in the lunate extending between the radiocarpal and midcarpal joints. The lunate fossa of the radius and the head of the capitate are normal. This condition is best managed with a proximal row carpectomy. These patients often do not do as

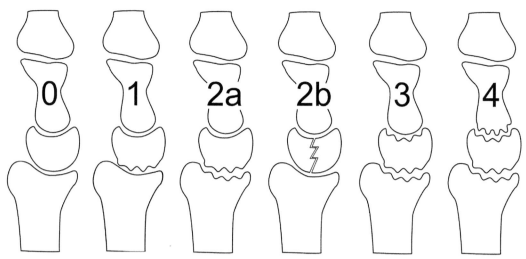

Fig. 4. Bain and Begg arthroscopic classification of Kienbock disease. The grade is determined by the number of nonfunctional articular surfaces. The grading system assist the surgeon to determine the best surgical option, based on the pathoanatomic findings. Although the classification was established based on arthroscopic finding, the grading can be determined based on imaging modalities. (*From* Bain GI, Begg M. Arthroscopic assessment and classification of Kienbock disease. Tech Hand Up Extrem Surg 2006;10(1):8–13; with permission.)

well with more complex procedures such as internal fixation or vascularized bone grafting.[9]

Grade 3

Three articular surfaces are nonfunctional.

Most likely it will be the capitate articular surface that remains functional. This situation could be managed with a hemiarthroplasty. Alternatively, until the results of hemiathroplasty have been established, a salvage procedure such as a total wrist fusion or arthroplasty could be performed.

Grade 4

All 4 articular surfaces are nonfunctional.

A total wrist fusion or arthroplasty is indicated.

When faced with a patient with Kienbock disease, the authors present the options of treatment, including nonoperative management. It is common to initially use a wrist splint and modification of activities. If the patient elects to proceed with surgery, the authors provide informed consent for the arthroscopy and the reconstruction procedure. The option of an isolated arthroscopy without a reconstructive procedure is usually performed in those patients with grade 0 or patients with advanced disease who did not want a full wrist fusion (eg, grade 3 or 4 Kienbock). In some cases, the consent includes proximal row carpectomy or radioscapholunate fusion.

The importance of the articular changes are better appreciated when they are seen as part of the overall pathologic process. The classification

and concepts presented in this article are pathoanatomic, and not just anatomic.

Pathologic phases of avascular necrosis

The authors consider that avascular necrosis should be considered as consisting of 3 pathologic phases: vascular (early), osseous (intermediate), and chondral (late) (**Fig. 5**).

1. Early vascular changes commence with ischemia, and subsequent necrosis and revascularization. Currently, the MRI and bone scan are of value in interpreting the vascular changes.
2. Intermediate osseous changes. Lichtman has described this well in the last 33 years. Quenzer and colleagues[11] reported on the value of the CT scan, and how it shows the detail of the osseous changes. The initial radiological changes are of sclerosis, followed by subchondral collapse.

It is the authors opinion that the subchondral bone plate is likely to be the critical part of the process of avascular necrosis, and that its survival is the key to the prognosis of articular cartilage, lunate, and the wrist. CT scanning can show the subchondral bone plate and assist in determining whether it is fragmented. The presence of a coronal fracture of the lunate is also well assessed on a CT scan. At arthroscopy, the articular cartilage can be palpated to determine whether there is a false floor. Arthroscopy assists in assessing the critical osseous structure of the lunate. Other chondral changes can be seen at arthroscopy.

Etiological Factors

Predisposed Individuals

Pathological Phases of AVN

1. Early – Vascular

2. Intermediate – Osseous

3. Late - Chondral

Fig. 5. The principle pathologic phases of avascular necrosis, showing the association between the vascular, osseous and chondral phases of Kienbock's Disease.

3. Late chondral changes. The changes identified are described earlier. The articular cartilage is often soft and can be indented, giving the impression that the articular surface has a false floor. This impression is in part caused by the arthroscopy being performed with traction on the wrist, so that the height of the lunate is artificially recreated. In the normally loaded Kienbock wrist, when the subchondral bone has collapsed, the body of the lunate is pressing directly onto the deep surface of the articular cartilage. With normal wrist function, this interface is subjected to considerable shear forces. Once the subchondral bone begins to fail, the shear forces tend to propagate parallel to the articular surface. The softness is most likely caused by loss of the subchondral bone. The authors postulate that it is the failure of the subchondral bone plate that is responsible for the failure to maintain the height of the lunate. Once the lunate articular cartilage has lost its

support, secondary changes are likely to occur quickly. We have witnessed that, once the proximal lunate articulation becomes non-functional, the lunate facet is usually also compromised.

The comments made earlier are the authors observations and recommendations. Regardless of the exact process, it is important to assess the articular surfaces involved and design the most appropriate procedure, taking into account the pathoanatomic findings identified.

The approach discussed in this paper respects the articular cartilage and places at the front of the decision-making process the pathoanatomic components of the articular cartilage in Kienbock avascular necrosis. It primarily respects the articular cartilage in the patient with avascular necrosis. This approach was developed for avascular necrosis of the lunate but, in principle, applies to other joints with avascular necrosis as well.

ACKNOWLEDGMENTS

We thank Robert Maurmo for assistance in the preparation of this manuscript.

REFERENCES

1. Irisarri C. Aetiology of Kienbocks disease. J Hand Surg 2004;29B(3):279–85.
2. Tsuge S, Nakamura R. Anatomical risk factors for Kienbock's disease. J Hand Surg Br 1993;18(1): 70–5.
3. Mirabello SC, Rosenthal DI, Smith RJ. Correlation of clinical and radiographic findings in Kienbock's disease. J Hand Surg Am 1987;12(6):1049–54.
4. Quenzer DE, Linscheid RL, Vidal MA, et al. Trispiral tomographic staging of Kienbock's disease. J Hand Surg Am 1997;22(3):396–403.
5. Ficat RP. Idiopathic bone necrosis of the femoral head. Early diagnosis and treatment. J Bone Joint Surg Br 1985;67(1):3–9.
6. Goldfarb CA, Hsu J, Gelberman RH, et al. The Lichtman classification for Kienbock's disease: an assessment of reliability. J Hand Surg Am 2003; 28(1):74–80.
7. Jafarnia K, Collins ED, Kohl HW 3rd, et al. Reliability of the Lichtman classification of Kienbock's disease. J Hand Surg Am 2000;25(3):529–34.
8. Menth-Chiari WA, Poehling GG, Wiesler ER, et al. Arthroscopic debridement for the treatment of Kienbock's disease. Arthroscopy 1999;15(1):12–9.
9. Bain GI, Begg M. Arthroscopic assessment and classification of Kienbock's disease. Tech Hand Up Extrem Surg 2006;10(1):8–13.

10. Bain GI, Richards RS, Roth JH. Wrist arthroscopy. In: Lichtman DM, Alexander AH, editors. The wrist and its disorders. 2 edition, vol 1. Philadelphia: W.B. Saunders; 1997.

11. Quenzer DE, Dobyns JH, Linscheid RL, et al. Radial recession osteotomy for Kienbock's disease. J Hand Surg Am 1997;22(3):386–95.

12. Lichtman DM, Mack GR, MacDonald RI, et al. Kienbock's disease: the role of silicone replacement arthroplasty. J Bone Joint Surg Am 1977;59(7):899–908.

13. Bain GI, Smith ML, Watts AC. Arthroscopic core decompression of the lunate in early stage Kienbocks disease of the lunate. Tech Hand Up Extrem Surg 2011;15(1):66–9.

Arthroscopic Management of Septic Arthritis of the Wrist

Douglas M. Sammer, MD[a], Alexander Y. Shin, MD[b],*

KEYWORDS

- Arthroscopy • Arthroscopic • Wrist • Septic arthritis
- Infection

Septic arthritis occurs in 2 to 5 per 100,000 individuals in the general population, but it is more common in certain groups (38 per 100,000 individuals with rheumatoid arthritis, and 70 per 100,000 individuals with a prosthetic joint).[1] Septic arthritis is a joint-threatening emergency and is associated with considerable morbidity and mortality.[2,3] Septic arthritis occurs in the lower extremity 80% of the time, and the most commonly involved joints are the knee (50%) and the hip (20%). When septic arthritis occurs in the upper extremity, it is estimated that 25% of cases involve the wrist.

Bacterial septic arthritis is classically divided into gonococcal and nongonococcal arthritis. In young sexually active individuals infected with *Neisseria gonorrhoeae*, this is a common cause of septic arthritis. However, outside of this population, *Staphylococcus aureus* is the most common causative organism.[4] Other organisms may also cause septic arthritis, including streptococcal species, gram-negative rods, mycobacteria, or fungal species. Septic arthritis is most commonly initiated by a hematogenous spread in patients with bacteremia, although direct joint inoculation from trauma or adjacent spread from a nearby infection, such as osteomyelitis, bursitis, or cellulitis, is also common.

Immunosuppression is an important risk factor for septic arthritis and is commonly seen in association with medications, such as disease-modifying antirheumatic drugs, corticosteroids, and chemotherapy; or with medical comorbidities, such as diabetes, HIV/AIDS, intravenous drug abuse, and end-stage renal disease. Increased patient age; the presence of a prosthetic joint; joint instrumentation; and any disease that affects the integrity of the articular surfaces, such as osteoarthritis, rheumatoid arthritis, and gout, are also risk factors.

DIAGNOSIS

The diagnosis of septic arthritis is made by history and physical examination and is supported by laboratory studies and imaging. Patients typically present with a swollen, erythematous, and painful joint with marked limitation of motion. Passive joint motion or axial loading of the joint is exquisitely painful. Systemic complaints include fever (90% of patients), chills, and sweats.[5] In cases of direct joint inoculation, there will be a history of surgery, recent joint injection, or penetrating injury. In cases of hematogenous spread, evidence of a distant infection, such as a urinary tract infection or endocarditis, should be sought.

Plain radiographs are generally nonspecific. They may be normal or show a widened joint space caused by effusion. Depending upon the duration of the septic arthritis, there may be joint space narrowing or destruction. In severe or untreated cases, there may be radiographic evidence of osteomyelitis. Osteoarthritis, rheumatoid arthritis, gout, and other arthritides are risk factors for septic arthritis, and changes consistent with chronic underlying arthritis are often seen in

Funding statement: No funding has been received related to this manuscript.
Financial disclosures: The authors have nothing to disclose.
[a] Department of Plastic Surgery, UT Southwestern Medical Center, 1801 Inwood Road, Dallas, TX 75390, USA
[b] Department of Orthopedic Surgery, Mayo Clinic, 200 First Street SW, Rochester, MN 55905, USA
* Corresponding author.
E-mail address: Shin.Alexander@Mayo.edu

Hand Clin 27 (2011) 331–334
doi:10.1016/j.hcl.2011.05.012
0749-0712/11/$ – see front matter © 2011 Elsevier Inc. All rights reserved.

patients with acute septic arthritis. Ultrasound and computed tomography scan are not particularly useful in the diagnosis of septic arthritis. Magnetic resonance imaging (MRI) may aid in differentiating between septic arthritis and transient aseptic synovitis of the hip in children, but it has not been demonstrated to be useful in diagnosing septic arthritis of the wrist. Appropriate treatment should not be delayed while awaiting an MRI in patients with suspected septic arthritis of the wrist.

Serology will often demonstrate leukocytosis (60% of patients), and an elevated erythrocyte sedimentation rate or C-reactive protein may be seen.[5,6] It should be noted, however, that the white blood cell (WBC) count may be normal or leucopenia may even be present in immunosuppressed patients.[7] Because other inflammatory processes, such as gout and rheumatoid arthritis, can mimic the history and findings of septic arthritis, arthrocentesis should be performed. Synovial fluid should be sent for gram stain, cultures, sensitivities (aerobic, anaerobic, fungal, and mycobacterial), cell count with differential, and crystal studies. A gram stain that is positive for organisms followed by a positive culture is confirmatory for septic arthritis. However, the gram stain is often negative in patients with septic arthritis, and cultures may not demonstrate a causative organism in up to 40% of cases.[2,8–10] The absence of crystals is supportive of the diagnosis of septic arthritis. However, gout and pseudogout are both risk factors for septic arthritis, and the presence of birefringent crystals does not rule out septic arthritis. With the exception of severely immunosuppressed patients, an elevated synovial fluid WBC count with left-shift (>75% neutrophils) is seen. A synovial WBC count of greater than 50,000 cells/mm^3 is considered highly suggestive of septic arthritis, and treatment should be initiated if the history and examination are consistent with septic arthritis. However, it should be noted that a synovial WBC count of greater than 50,000 cells/mm^3 can be seen with other diseases, such as gout, and a synovial WBC count of less than 50,000 cells/mm^3 may be seen in up to one-third of patients with confirmed septic arthritis.[11]

TREATMENT

Effective treatment of septic arthritis involves emergent irrigation and debridement (I&D) of the joint, combined with appropriate intravenous antibiotics. In the wrist, I&D is commonly performed in an open fashion.[8,12,13] However, in other joints, such as the knee, hip, and shoulder, arthroscopic I&D of septic arthritis is well described.[14–18] There are several potential advantages to arthroscopic

I&D of the wrist, including smaller incisions, limited disruption of the dorsal wrist ligaments and capsule, less pain, superior visualization of the articular surfaces, and no open contaminated wound requiring dressing changes. Furthermore, a recent study by Sammer and Shin[7] provides evidence that arthroscopic I&D may be associated with fewer operations and shorter hospital stays in patients with isolated septic arthritis of the wrist.

In this study, patients with septic arthritis of the wrist treated by open or arthroscopic I&D over an 11-year period at a single institution were reviewed. The primary outcome measurements were the number of I&Ds required to treat the infection, the length of hospital stay (LOS), and perioperative mortality. Thirty-six patients (40 wrists) were included in the study. Seventeen patients (19 wrists) were treated with open I&D, and 19 patients (21 wrists) were treated arthroscopically. Overall, there was no difference between the open and arthroscopic cohorts in terms of the number of I&Ds required to treat the infection or the hospital LOS. However, when the investigators evaluated patients with isolated septic arthritis of the wrist, and excluded patients with multiple sites of infection, a significant difference between the two cohorts was found. Patients who underwent open I&D required an average of 3 operations to successfully treat the infection, whereas patients who underwent arthroscopic I&D were all successfully treated with a single operation ($p = .001$). Furthermore, those who underwent open I&D had an average hospital LOS of 16 days, compared with 6 days for those treated arthroscopically ($p = .04$). Ninety-day perioperative mortality was high in both groups: 18% in the open cohort and 21% in the arthroscopic cohort.

ARTHROSCOPIC IRRIGATION AND DEBRIDEMENT

Although arthroscopic I&D can be performed for most cases of septic arthritis of the wrist, several contraindications exist. Postoperative wrist infections usually require open I&D because the infection involves not only the joint but also the soft-tissue planes and any hardware, fracture, or osteotomy that may be present. Prior incisions and scarring make arthroscopy more difficult and are a relative contraindication. Osteomyelitis is also a relative contraindication. Although small areas of osteomyelitis can be debrided arthroscopically if they are accessible from the joint, more extensive osteomyelitis requires open debridement. In addition, some wrist joints are inaccessible with an arthroscope, either because of small size (such as that of an infant or small child) or because of severe joint destruction, and the I&D should be performed in an open fashion. Finally, purulence that extends outside of the radiocarpal and midcarpal joints (for example within the dorsal subcutaneous tissue) is an indication for open I&D.

Arthroscopic I&D is performed with patients under general anesthesia to avoid regional block injections in the setting of an upper-extremity infection. Patients are placed supine, with the shoulder abducted 90° and the elbow flexed 90° on the hand table. Intravenous antibiotics are administered only if synovial fluid has already been sent for cultures. If not, antibiotics are withheld until intraoperative cultures have been taken. A pneumatic tourniquet is placed on the arm, and the upper extremity is prepped and draped sterilely. An arthroscopy traction tower is placed on the hand table and secured. The hand is then suspended from the tower with finger traps from the index and middle fingers. The forearm is stabilized to the vertical bar of the tower in neutral rotation, and the arm is secured to the hand table and base of the tower with straps. It is important to use appropriate padding. 4.5 to 6.8 kg of traction are applied through the traction tower. A gravity inflow irrigation system of 3 L of normal saline is hung from an intravenous pole. It is critical to use gravity inflow rather than a mechanical pump in the setting of septic arthritis to avoid extravasation of infected fluid. A 2.7-mm, 30° angled arthroscope is assembled with the light source and camera. A 2.0- or 2.9-mm full-radius joint shaver with suction is assembled.

If arthrocentesis was not performed preoperatively, it is performed before arthroscopy. A sterile 18-gauge needle is inserted into the radiocarpal joint, and synovial fluid is aspirated. This procedure is repeated at the midcarpal joint if required to obtain an adequate sample. Synovial fluid is sent for gram stain, aerobic, anaerobic, acid-fast bacillus, and fungal cultures and sensitivities. If there is enough fluid, it is sent for quantitative cell counts and crystal studies. Intravenous antibiotics are now administered. Before the arthroscopy portals are developed, anatomic landmarks are marked, including the Lister tubercle, the dorsal margin of the radius and ulna, the radial styloid, the distal radioulnar joint, and the course of the extensor tendons. This procedure may be occasionally difficult secondary to the soft-tissue swelling. Fluoroscopy can be of assistance in determining portal placement. The 3-4, 4-5, radial midcarpal, and ulnar midcarpal portals are marked. Each portal consists of a longitudinal incision 5 mm in length. The 3-4 portal is located approximately 1 cm distal to the Lister tubercle, between the extensor pollicis longus and extensor

digitorum communis tendons. The 4-5 portal is between the extensor digitorum communis and extensor digiti quinti tendons, approximately 1 cm ulnar to the 3-4 portal. Because of the radial inclination of the radius, the 3-4 portal will be slightly more distal than the 4-5 portal. Next, the midcarpal portals are marked. The radial midcarpal portal is 1 cm distal to the 3-4 portal, in line with the radial border of the third ray. The ulnar midcarpal portal is 1 cm distal to the 4-5 portal. After marking, the arm is elevated for 1 minute before the tourniquet is elevated to 250 mm Hg. Alternatively, an Esmarch dressing can be used from the mid forearm proximal for exsanguination of the arm. Skin-only incisions are made with a number-11 blade. A small curved hemostat is used to spread through the soft tissue down to the joint capsule, preserving the superficial sensory nerves and veins. The wrist capsule is entered by applying gentle pressure with a blunt trocar. For the 3-4 portal, the trocar is angled 11° proximally to parallel the articular surface. At the 4-5 portal, the angle of entry is neutral. At the midcarpal portals, the trocar is also angled proximally because of the shape of the midcarpal joint. The blunt trocar, cannula, and inflow irrigation tubing are assembled and are inserted into the 3-4 portal. The trocar is removed from the cannula, and the arthroscope is inserted through the cannula. The motorized joint shaver is introduced through the 4-5 portal. Gravity inflow is started, and outflow is provided with low suction through the joint shaver. Joint surfaces are examined for signs of cartilage damage. The interosseous ligaments are examined for tears, widening, step-offs, and laxity, and the integrity of the radiocarpal ligaments is examined. Next, the triangular fibrocartilaginous complex on the ulnar side of the wrist is evaluated. Synovitis, purulence, and loculations are often encountered during arthroscopy for septic arthritis, and they are debrided with the joint shaver. Photographs are taken to document the quality of the articular surfaces and the presence of synovitis, loculations, and debris. Once the joint has been explored and debrided, the suction on the joint shaver is turned to high, and the joint is irrigated with the remainder of the 3 L of irrigation fluid. This procedure is accomplished quickly by using gravity inflow through the cannula at the 3-4 portal and suction outflow through the shaver. Next, attention is turned to the midcarpal joint. The assembled trocar and cannula with attached inflow tubing are inserted into the radial midcarpal portal. The trocar is removed, and the arthroscope is inserted through the cannula. The joint shaver is introduced through the ulnar midcarpal portal. The same process of debridement and inspection is performed from the midcarpal joint. The midcarpal joint is then irrigated with 3 L of irrigation fluid. All instruments are withdrawn, and the finger traps and the traction tower are removed from the field. The skin incisions are left open. The wrist is immobilized in 20° of extension with a well-padded plaster splint.

SUMMARY

Septic arthritis of the wrist is a joint-threatening emergency that is associated with substantial morbidity and mortality and requires urgent I&D. Historically, I&D of the wrist has been performed in an open fashion. However, there are several potential advantages to arthroscopic I&D of the wrist, including smaller incisions, better visualization of the articular surfaces, and no large, contaminated soft-tissue wound requiring dressing changes. Furthermore, there is evidence that in patients with isolated septic arthritis of the wrist, arthroscopic I&D results in fewer operations and shorter hospital stays.

REFERENCES

1. Ho G, Jue SJ, Cook PP. Arthritis caused by bacteria or their components. In: Harris ED, Budd RC, Firestein GS, et al, editors. Kelley's textbook of rheumatology. Philadelphia: Elsevier; 2005.
2. Mehta P, Schnall SB, Zalavras CG. Septic arthritis of the shoulder, elbow, and wrist. Clin Orthop Relat Res 2006;451:42–5.
3. Shirtliff ME, Mader JT. Acute septic arthritis. Clin Microbiol Rev 2002;15(4):527–44.
4. Smith JW, Piercy EA. Infectious arthritis. Clin Infect Dis 1995;20(2):225–30. [quiz: 231].
5. Goldenberg DL, Cohen AS. Acute infectious arthritis. A review of patients with nongonococcal joint infections (with emphasis on therapy and prognosis). Am J Med 1976;60(3):369–77.
6. Weston VC, Jones AC, Bradbury N, et al. Clinical features and outcome of septic arthritis in a single UK health district 1982–1991. Ann Rheum Dis 1999;58(4):214–9.
7. Sammer DM, Shin AY. Comparison of arthroscopic and open treatment of septic arthritis of the wrist. J Bone Joint Surg Am 2009;91(6):1387–93.
8. Meier R, Lanz U. [Septic arthritis of the wrist]. Handchir Mikrochir Plast Chir 2007;39(2):112–7 [in German].
9. Kim SJ, Choi NH, Ko SH, et al. Arthroscopic treatment of septic arthritis of the hip. Clin Orthop Relat Res 2003;(407):211–4.
10. Thiery JA. Arthroscopic drainage in septic arthritides of the knee: a multicenter study. Arthroscopy 1989;5(1):65–9.
11. Li SF, Henderson J, Dickman E, et al. Laboratory tests in adults with monoarticular arthritis: can they rule out a septic joint? Acad Emerg Med 2004;11(3):276–80.
12. Rashkoff ES, Burkhalter WE, Mann RJ. Septic arthritis of the wrist. J Bone Joint Surg Am 1983;65(6):824–8.
13. Stevanovic MV, Sharpe F. Acute infections in the hand. In: Green DP, Hotchkiss RN, Pederson WC, et al, editors. Green's operative hand surgery. Philadelphia: Elsevier; 2005. p. 55–93.
14. Balabaud L, Gaudras J, Boeri C, et al. Results of treatment of septic knee arthritis: a retrospective series of 40 cases. Knee Surg Sports Traumatol Arthrosc 2007;15(4):387–92.
15. Jarrett MP, Grossman L, Sadler AH, et al. The role of arthroscopy in the treatment of septic arthritis. Arthritis Rheum 1981;24(5):737–9.
16. Jeon IH, Choi CH, Seo JS, et al. Arthroscopic management of septic arthritis of the shoulder joint. J Bone Joint Surg Am 2006;88(8):1802–6.
17. Nusem I, Jabur MK, Playford EG. Arthroscopic treatment of septic arthritis of the hip. Arthroscopy 2006; 22(8):902.e1–3.
18. Sanchez AA, Hennrikus WL. Arthroscopically assisted treatment of acute septic knees in infants using the micro-joint arthroscope. Arthroscopy 1997; 13(3):350–4.

Dry Arthroscopy and its Applications

Francisco del Piñal, MD, DrMed

KEYWORDS

- Dry arthroscopy • Wrist arthroscopy
- Arthroscopic technique • Clinical applications

Arthroscopy traditionally has been performed using fluid to create a working cavity ("wet" arthroscopy). Distending the joint with fluid, however, is not nuisance free. Fluid infiltrates tissues, escapes through the portals, and might cause serious problems such as compartment syndrome. Fluid enormously hampers any concomitant surgery after the arthroscopic exploration, due to loss of definition of anatomic planes. Finally, the use of fluid makes it impossible to combine arthroscopy with semi-open procedures such as intra-articular osteotomies and triangular fibrocartilage (TFC) reinsertions, as massive seepage of fluid will cause constant loss of vision.

Extrapolating that in other "scopies" in the human body, such as laparoscopy or thoracoscopy, fluid was not used to maintain the optic cavity, the author realized that traction through the fingers was sufficient to keep the wrist cavity open, making the use of fluid unnecessary. In fact, all the aforementioned inconveniencies could be circumvented, without modifying the visual properties, if fluid were not infused inside the joint ("dry" arthroscopy).[1] Large portals/mini incisions can be created for the passage of large instruments or the extraction of large bony fragments, without fear of losing fluid tightness. Open and semi-open arthroscopic assisted procedures can hence be easily combined. Finally, traditional open surgery can be performed immediately after the arthroscopy exploration, leaving tissue in pristine condition, as there has been no extravasation of fluid outside the capsule (**Fig. 1**).

Not using fluid, on the other hand, engenders a new set of problems secondary to loss of vision caused by splashes on the tip of the scope or blood and debris in the joint. This situation may induce the novice to give up at the first difficulty met, but the advantages of the dry technique far outweigh the difficulties encountered on the learning curve. In this work the technical tips to carry out an uneventful operation are presented in detail.

SURGICAL TECHNIQUE

The "dry" arthroscopy technique is similar to a standard wrist arthroscopy ("wet"), except for that fluid is not used to maintain the optic cavity. As stated, the main shortcoming comes from the fact that if one is not able to get rid of the blood and splashes that obscure vision in an expeditious manner, surgery will become a torment and one will give up on the dry technique.

Intuitively, one would think that removing the scope and wiping off the lens with a wet sponge is a good way of clearing the visual field. Although effective, this maneuver is time consuming and, in a fracture or other complex procedures described in this article, there may be so much blood or debris that the maneuver may need to be repeated an exasperating number of times. Based on his experience with more than 700 dry wrist arthroscopies, and—more importantly—seeing how others in the laboratory and surgery struggle with the same difficulties over and over again, the author can recommend the following tips that are critical for a smooth procedure, some of which are improvements on the previous publication.[1]

- The valve of the sheath of the scope should be kept open at all times to allow the air to circulate freely inside the joint. Otherwise, either the suction of the shaver will not

Unit of Hand-Wrist and Plastic Surgery, Hospital Mutua Montañesa, Instituto de Cirugía Plástica y de la Mano, Calderón de la Barca 16-entlo, E- 39002-Santander, Spain
E-mail address: drpinal@drpinal.com

Hand Clin 27 (2011) 335–345
doi:10.1016/j.hcl.2011.05.011
0749-0712/11/$ – see front matter © 2011 Elsevier Inc. All rights reserved.

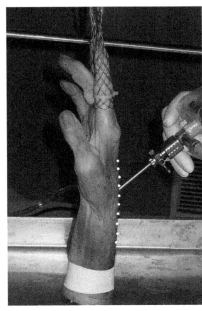
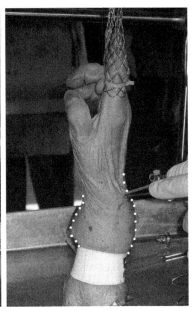

Fig. 1. The deformity of the wrist due to fluid extravasation after 1 hour of wet arthroscopy (*right*) as compared with the left, which was operated on for the same amount of time but under the dry technique. Pictures were taken during a teaching course with cadavers in Strasbourg. Both were operated by students simultaneously in different working posts. (Copyright Francisco del Piñal, MD, 2010.)

function properly or the capsule will collapse inwards because of the power of the suction, resulting in blocked vision. This aspect is critical and cannot be overemphasized (**Fig. 2**).

- Suction is necessary to clear the field but, paradoxically, suction might also blur the vision by stirring up the contents of the joint (debris, blood or remaining saline) that may stick to the tip of the scope. It is critical,

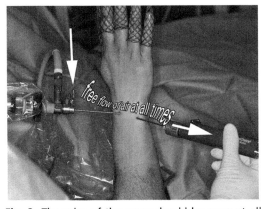

Fig. 2. The valve of the scope should be open at all times so as to allow air to circulate freely. (*From* del Piñal F. Treatment of explosion-type distal radius fractures. In: del Piñal F, Mathoulin C, Luchetti C, editors. Arthroscopic management of distal radius fractures. Berlin: Springer Verlag; 2010. p. 41–65; with permission.)

therefore, to open the suction of the shaver or burr only when there is the need to aspirate something. Suction power should be locked when not needed. To sum up, the valve of the sheath of the scope should be open at all times, but suction should only be used as needed.

- Avoid getting too close with the tip of the scope when working with burrs or osteotomes, to avert splashes that might block your vision. Minor splashes can be removed by gently rubbing the tip of scope on the local soft tissue (capsule, fat, and so forth).
- When a clear field is needed, so as to see a gap or a step-off, the author used to recommend drying out the joint with neurosurgical patties.[1] However, the author rarely resorts to this technique now, and prefers to connect a syringe with 5 to 10 mL of saline to the side valve of the scope and then aspirate it with an arthroscopic shaver, to get rid of blood and debris. Pressure on the plunger of the syringe is unnecessary, as the negative pressure exerted by the shaver will suck the saline into the joint, thus preventing any extravasation (**Fig. 3**). Once all the fluid has been aspirated the syringe is removed, and again the suction power of the shaver is enough to dry out the joint sufficiently, thus allowing the surgeon to work. This maneuver should be

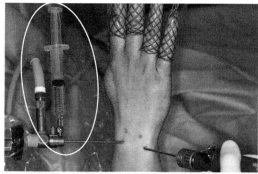
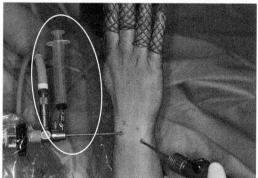

Fig. 3. Method used to wash out the joint and clear it of blood. Notice that the negative pressure exerted by the shaver is sufficient to aspirate the saline without extravasation of fluid. (*From* del Piñal F. Treatment of explosion-type distal radius fractures. In: del Piñal F, Mathoulin C, Luchetti C, editors. Arthroscopic management of distal radius fractures. Berlin: Springer Verlag; 2010. p. 41–65; with permission.)

repeated as necessary throughout the procedure, as it is much quicker than struggling with blood in the joint, or trying to dry it out with the patties.

- An important waste of time occurs when the full-radius resector, burr, or any other instruments connected to a suction machine clog because the aspirated debris dries out. When this happens the operation has to be temporarily halted to dismount and irrigate the full-radius resector for dislodging the debris. This situation is to be avoided at all costs by clearing the tubing with periodic saline aspiration from an external basin by the operating-room nurse, or by the surgeon through joint irrigation. Joint flushing should also be done in a systematic fashion in some procedures, such as intercarpal arthrodesis or arthroscopic proximal carpectomy, in which prolonged use of the full-radius resectors and burrs may cause heating of the instrument itself, causing local burns (see later discussion).

- Finally, one must understand that at most times vision will never be completely clear but still sufficient to safely accomplish the goals of the procedure. Having a completely dried field except for at specific times during the procedure is unnecessary and wastes valuable time, and the author relies more on the irrigation-suction explained above.

The technique can be summarized in these 3 fundamental tips:

- The valve of the scope should be open at all times
- The suction should be closed except when needed
- The joint should be irrigated as needed to remove debris and blood.

CONTRAINDICATIONS

The dry technique is contraindicated when using thermal probes, lasers, and so forth, as the heat generated will not dissipate, risking widespread cartilage damage. The problem is solved easily, however, by swapping to the "wet" technique during the specific moment that these kinds of instruments are being used. Once the thermal shrinkage or debridement is finished, the saline is disconnected and air allowed to flow in the joint. The remaining fluid is sucked out with the full-radius resector and the procedure continues "dry." In very special scenarios where running fluid is paramount, such as in septic arthritis, the use of the dry technique will offer no advantage and is not advised.

Risk of compartment syndrome has been considered a contraindication for arthroscopy, particularly after severe fractures, but this is not a problem when using the dry technique. Furthermore, open wounds are not considered a contraindication of the dry arthroscopy either, provided debridement of the portal is carried out and thorough irrigation of the joint is performed at the end of the procedure.

One concern of surgeons regarding dry arthroscopy is the possibility of thermal damage inside the joint by the tip of the scope. In the author's experience this has never occurred, as the tip of the scope never warms up to that point. The reader should be warned, however, that the author has experienced minor contact burns at the portals and the dorsal skin, by the full-radius resector and burr. The rotating mechanism of these instruments heats up, as a result of friction, when used for very long periods of time. This overheating is easily overcome by flushing the joint with saline that will cool down the full-radius resector, and also will improve vision.

CLINICAL APPLICATIONS

The author uses the dry technique in nearly all has arthroscopic explorations, as he personally has not found it necessary to use vaporizers. There are, however, 4 common scenarios for which not using fluid makes an enormous difference, namely, TFC-complex reattachments, distal radius fractures and malunions, and arthroscopic arthrodeses. Because the first one is covered in another article by Yao and colleagues elsewhere in this issue, the focus here is on the technical aspects of the latter 3 scenarios.

Distal Radius Fractures and Malunions

Despite the existence in the literature of well-performed Level I studies[2–4] supporting the use of the arthroscope when dealing with articular distal radius fractures, there is general resistance in the Hand Surgeon community to admit so. This standpoint is sometimes justified as being due to the very small risk of compartment syndrome, and more so to the massive swelling that accompanies the wet arthroscopy that makes the open part of the procedure more awkward. Although the latter reason is true, the unvoiced reason lies in the technical difficulties of the arthroscopic part itself. This is more so the more comminuted the fracture is, which paradoxically is the one type that benefits most from having an arthroscopic assisted reduction.[5] Yet there is no other single field in wrist arthroscopy where the dry technique can make such a huge difference and ease the procedure, as when dealing with articular fractures of the wrist. The dry arthroscopy allows an unimpeded combination between the open-fixation part and the ability to watch the cartilaginous reduction as well as assess ligamentous and TFC injuries.

The author's current technique[6,7] includes the use of volar locking plates in combination with arthroscopy, except in some specific fractures, such as radial styloid, where cannulated screws through a transverse incision in the styloid is the preferred fixation method. For the typical 3-part or 4-part fracture, the radius is approached between the flexor carpi ulnaris (FCR) and the radial artery. After a preliminary reduction, a volar locking plate is applied and stabilized by inserting only the screw into the elliptical hole on the stem of the plate. The articular fragments are reduced to the plate, which acts as a mold, and once the "best" reduction is obtained as judged by fluoroscopic views, the articular fragments are secured to the plate by inserting Kirschner wires (K-wire) through the distal K-wire holes in the plate. It should be underscored that definitive fixation (screws or pegs) should not yet be used, as any change will not be possible later.

The hand is suspended from a bow, the fingers pointing to the ceiling, with a customized system that allows easy connection and disconnection from the bow without losing sterility, as fluoroscopic checkups are needed.[8] Traction is applied to all of the fingers with countertraction of 7 to 10 kg. A small transverse incision is made just distal to Lister's tubercle and, after dilating the portal with a straight mosquito, the scope (2.7 mm; 30° angle) is introduced and directed ulnarly. In the swollen wrist, it may be very difficult to establish a 6R portal, more so because the TFC may be detached from the fovea, acting as a lid blocking the entrance into the radiocarpal joint. This eventuality is overcome through establishing this portal by going blindly with a hemostat in a radial direction immediately radial to the extensor carpi ulnaris, just brushing past the proximal triquetrum.

The blood and debris are aspirated by a 2.9-mm shaver inserted in the 6R. Flushing and debridement is performed until the joint is completely clean. Once the elements that need to be mobilized are identified, the scope is swapped to the 6R, where it will stay until the entire fixation is done. In this position, on top of the ulnar head, the scope will have a steady point to rest on, and will not impede reduction or displace reduced fragments (**Fig. 4**).

In simpler cases where only a single fragment remains unreduced, the fragment is freed by backing out the specific K-wire that kept it secured to the plate. Depressed fragments are lifted by hooking them with the tip of a shoulder or knee arthroscopy probe introduced from portal 3–4 (**Fig. 5**).

Elevated fragments nearly always correspond to rim fragments that, due to the effect of traction, are overdistracted. These fragments are easily repositioned by the assistant decreasing traction while the surgeon levels them with the probe or a Freer elevator. Once the fragment is reduced, it is held in position with a bone tenaculum, and stabilized by pushing the corresponding K-wire through the K-wire holes in the plate again. Free osteochondral fragments are extremely unstable, and when repositioned sink into the metaphyseal void. To avoid this the author creates a supporting hammock where they can lie. The distal layer of pegs is inserted in the plate, while keeping these fragments slightly overreduced. Then they are impacted by using a Freer elevator or by releasing the traction and using the corresponding carpal bone as a mold. A grasper can be useful to grab and twist a severely displaced fragment.[7]

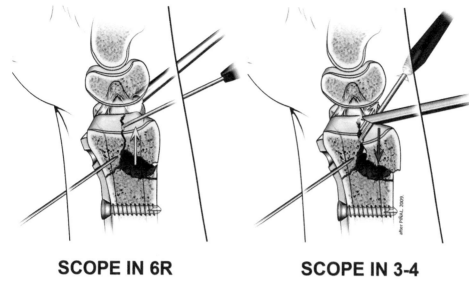

SCOPE IN 6R   SCOPE IN 3-4

Fig. 4. If the scope is placed in 6R it will rest on top of the ulnar head providing a stable platform from which to work, thus avoiding conflict with the reduction (*left*). Instability of the scope and conflict of space during the reduction (*yellow and red arrows*) is inevitable when the scope is placed in any other portal (*right*). (Copyright Francisco del Piñal, MD, 2010.)

Still under arthroscopic control, locking pegs/screws are inserted in the plate by the other surgeon in critical spots, so as to make the articular surface stable to probe palpation. This part of the operation is awkward because the flexor tendons are in tension, blocking the vision of the plate. Retracting the tendons ulnarwards with a Farabeuf and reducing the traction to release the flexor tendons may ease the task. As soon as the major articular fragments are stabilized, the hand is placed flat on the operating table, as in this position the remaining pegs and screws can be inserted expeditiously (**Fig. 6**).

Only in the most comminuted cases will several fragments continue to be displaced after the fluoroscopic part of the operation. Backing out all the K-wires, and attempting to reduce and fix all fragments at the same time, is an impossible

endeavor. The author recommends a step-by-step procedure beginning preferably from the ulnar part of the radius, advancing in a radial direction. The mechanics of the procedure are similar as for a single fragment: the corresponding K-wire is backed out, the fragment reduced, and the K-wire pushed in, building up the rest of the articular surface on this foundation.

Once the radius fixation is over, the hand is again placed on traction, and the distal radioulnar joint and midcarpal joint are assessed for instability or ligament damage.

Arthroscopic Guided Osteotomy for Distal Radius Malunion

Arthroscopy can be invaluable to locate step-offs, to visualize the geometry of the malunited

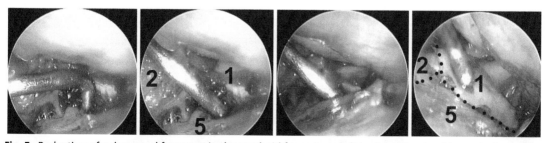

Fig. 5. Reduction of a depressed fragment in the scaphoid fossa. From left to right: the shoulder probe is gauging the step-off (3 mm), hooking the depressed fragment, elevating it, and leveling it to the rest of the joint. Scope in 6R, viewing radially in a right wrist. 1, volar rim of the scaphoid fossa; 2, dorsal rim; 5, scaphoid fossa. (Copyright Francisco del Piñal, MD, 2010.)

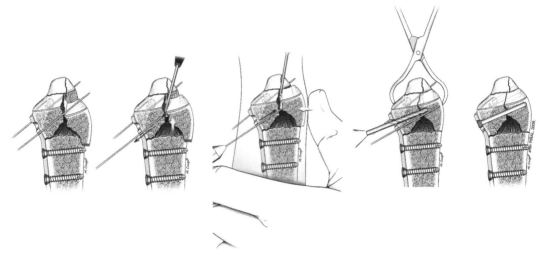

Fig. 6. Summary of the author's technique to reduce and stabilize the common scenario of a posterior depressed fragment that remains unreduced. Notice that the K-wire is backed out sufficiently enough to release this malpositioned fragment, while the rest of the reduction remains unaffected during the whole maneuver. (Copyright Francisco del Piñal, MD, 2010.)

fragment, to osteotomize the bone precisely at the interface between the malunited fragment and the articular surface, and to assess the reduction (**Fig. 7**). In fact this is more so, as fluoroscopy has not proved very reliable even in the setting of acute fractures,[9,10] and because performing the osteotomy blindly can section the joint surface in an undesired spot.[11]

The technique of osteotomy has been described previously,[8,11] and the early results reported.[12] In brief, the procedure is started by preparing the proposed site of plate fixation with the arm lying on the hand table. To facilitate the separation of the fragments when later doing the intra-articular osteotomy, the external callus is removed with a rongeur and the outer callus is weakened with an osteotome. No attempt is made to go all the way to the joint or to do any rough bending or prying

open of the fragment with the osteotome, as this may break the cartilage at the incorrect place. A plate, when needed, is preplaced at this stage, and held in position with a single proximal screw as explained for acute fractures. The hand is then placed in traction. An arthroscopic arthrolysis is first performed to create working space, as the joint is scarred and unyielding. For cutting the bone the author uses a shoulder periosteal elevator (of 15° and 30° angle) (Arthrex AR-1342-30° and AR-1342-15°; Arthrex, Naples, FL, USA), and also straight and curved osteotomes (Arthrex AR-1770 and AR-1771). Instruments with different angles are required to avoid damaging the cartilage, and laceration of the extensor tendons are to be avoided by the appropriate technique.[11] The osteotomes also have to be inserted through different portals to adapt to the different configurations of

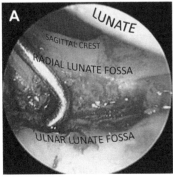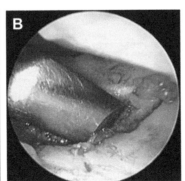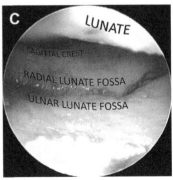

Fig. 7. (*A*) Correction of a 4-mm step-off on the lunate fossa (right wrist scope in 6R). (*B*) The osteotome (entering the joint through a dorsal portal) is separating the malunited fragments. (*C*) Corresponding view after reduction. (Copyright Francisco del Piñal, MD, 2010.)

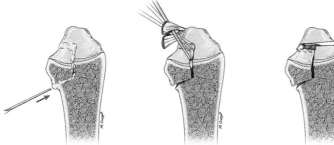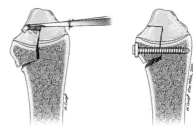

Fig. 8. Most malunions require multiple accesses and combinations of osteotomy types. Notice that the osteotome is introduced into the cleft between the radioscaphocapitate and long radiolunate ligaments when using the volar-radial portal. (Copyright Francisco del Piñal, MD, 2010.)

the fracture (**Fig. 8**). Stabilization of the fragments is performed with volar locking plates when several fragments are mobilized; screws or buttressing plates are used when only one fragment needs to be addressed.

Arthroscopic Arthrodesis

Intercarpal or radiocarpal arthrodesis can be performed arthroscopically.[13] Some may view this with skepticism, but the procedure is sound not only because there will be a cosmetic benefit,

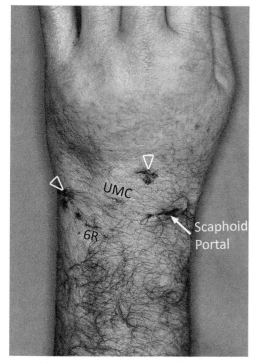

Fig. 9. The incisions required for a 4CF are shown in this patient. Hollowed arrows point to the entrance of the cannulated screws. Notice the minimal swelling 3 days after the procedure with the dry arthroscopy. (Copyright Francisco del Piñal, MD, 2010.)

but above all because the degree of insult to the wrist ligaments will be minimized. Ligament preservation will keep the blood supply to the bones intact, with less scarring to the capsule, promoting in turn bony healing and less stiffness, respectively. The operation as described by Ho[133] using a "wet" technique is very cumbersome, due to fluid escaping through the portals and to the difficulty in maintaining the bone graft in the proper position. Furthermore, because the operation takes a long time the amount of tissue infiltration becomes massive, which is detrimental at the time of fixation.

The dry technique can be invaluable in this complicated operation, which ranks among the most difficult procedures in wrist arthroscopy. Several factors contribute to this complexity: the anatomy is distorted; it takes considerable time to burr out and to match the bone surfaces for arthrodesis; there is a need for bone graft insertion; and finally, the surgeon has to "blindly" insert the guidewires for the cannulated screws. All these steps are greatly facilitated if the tissues are not infiltrated. If the dry technique is used, all bony landmarks will be recognizable by palpation throughout the operation.

The aim of this work is not to present in detail any of the techniques; however, a brief description, using the 4-corner fusion (4CF) as a reference, helps to highlight the advantages of the dry technique. The procedure commences by creating the portals, which are easily made ulnarly (6R and ulnar midcarpal portal). With advanced scapholunate advance collapse (SLAC) or scaphoid nonunion advanced collapse (SNAC), the radial portals are more difficult to establish, because of architectural derangement of the carpus and, often, scarring from previous surgery. The author's preference is to create a large (1.5-cm) transverse "scaphoid portal" (midway between 3–4 and radial midcarpal portal) corresponding to the location of the scapholunate gap or the scaphoid nonunion

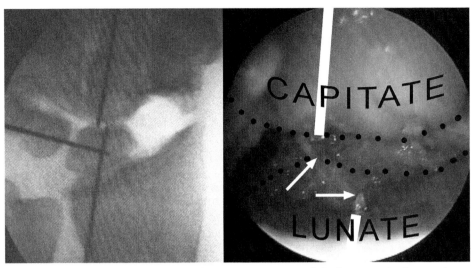

Fig. 10. Fluoroscopic and arthroscopic control of the correct position of the lunate on its fossa and good alignment of the capitolunate guidewire are paramount for a good outcome. Arrows point to the tips of the radiolunate and capitolunate wires, while white strips mimic the wires' path in the bones. (Copyright Francisco del
Piñal, MD, 2010.)

(**Fig. 9**). From there, work can be performed in both
the radiocarpal and midcarpal directions.

One begins by inserting the scope in 6R and
locating the "scaphoid portal" with a needle. An
aggressive 2.9-mm full-radius resector is inserted
through this portal. Hypertrophic synovium, bone
debris, and scarred tissue in the dorsal capsule
are radically resected to create a larger working
space. As soon as possible one switches to
a 4.5-mm full-radius resector, to speed up the
process. In both dry and wet techniques, one of
the difficulties arises from the need to deal with
a large quantity of bone debris secondary to
scaphoid and/or subchondral bone excision. As
explained in the section on surgical technique,
during burring the suction should be switched off
to maintain good vision, and irrigation-suction
should be intermittently used to remove debris.

In the best of circumstances, burring out the whole
scaphoid with a 4.5-mm (or even a 5.5-mm) burr is
time consuming. For this reason, whenever
possible, the author tries to remove a large part
of the scaphoid in one piece after releasing it
from the soft tissue connections with a banana
blade or a full-radius resector. In 4CF one can be
quite rough, for the sake of speediness, in the
radial side of the joint, with osteotomes and burrs;
denting the cartilage of the radial surface of the
capitate, proximal trapezium, and trapezoid is
inconsequential, as all this area will be a void at
the end of the operation. Similarly, the scaphoid
fossa will be nonarticulating, and as a matter of
fact a moderate styloidectomy is always needed.

After the scaphoid has been removed (piecemeal,
or burred out), the cartilage and hard subchondral
bone of the joints to be arthrodesed are resected

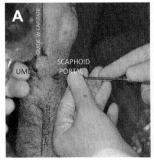
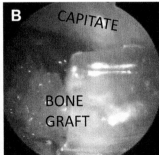
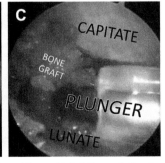

Fig. 11. Intraoperative view while the bone graft is being delivered in the midcarpal joint through the "scaphoid
portal." (*A*) The surgeon is holding the cannula with the left hand and the plunger (the scope sheath) with the
right hand. (*B, C*) Corresponding arthroscopic view while the bone graft is being delivered in the midcarpal joint
by pushing the bone graft into the joint by the plunger. (Copyright Francisco del Piñal, MD, 2010.)

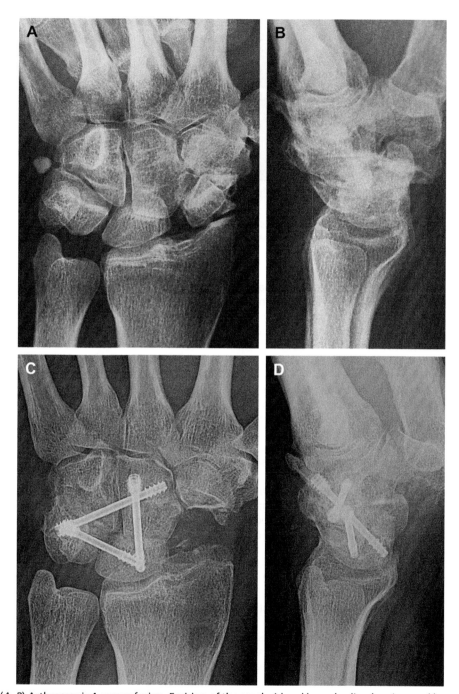

Fig. 12. (*A, B*) Arthroscopic 4-corner fusion. Excision of the scaphoid and loose bodies, burring, and bone grafting were all done arthroscopically. Protected range of motion was started 2 weeks after the operation. (*C, D*) Solid bony healing at 9 weeks. (Copyright Francisco del Piñal, MD, 2010.)

until healthy cancellous bone is exposed. For this step the author prefers pineapple-shaped, rather than ball-shaped, burrs. The latter tend to produce "holes" instead of an even surface, and easily get "caught" (snagged or stuck). Again for the sake of

speediness, 4.5-mm diameter burrs are preferred if space permits.

Once the bony surfaces are prepared for arthrodeses, the hand is taken off from traction and the position of the lunate assessed. Usually

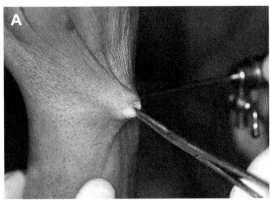
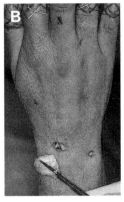
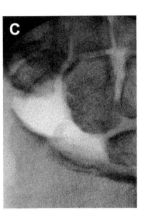

Fig. 13. (*A, B*) The proximal pole of the scaphoid is being "delivered" in one piece through the "scaphoid portal" during an arthroscopic assisted proximal row carpectomy (*B*). (*C*) The distal pole was burred out. (Copyright Francisco del Piñal, MD, 2010.)

the lunate is dorsiflexed and translocated ulnarly, and needs to be reduced in neutral in the lunate fossa; this is achieved by the surgeon maximally flexing the wrist and at the same time translocating the wrist radially. A K-wire inserted about 2 cm proximal to portal 4–5 and directed slightly radially will hit the lunate on its center.

The joints to be fixed are now temporarily stabilized in the reduced position with the guidewires for the cannulated screws. In the author's view this is the trickiest part of the whole operation, as the screws should sit in an exact position to achieve good purchase and avoid screw collision. Apart from the fluoroscopic aid it is crucial, for orientation purposes, to palpate all the bony landmarks. This task becomes a very difficult in a swollen wrist, just as when the "wet" technique is used. Three cannulated screws are used: one capitolunate, one triquetrolunate, and the last a triquetrocapitate. The capitate-lunate screw is directed from the dorsal and distal aspect of the capitate to volar-proximal on the lunate. The triquetrum-lunate screw is directed from volarly in the triquetrum to dorsally in the lunate. The triquetrum-capitate screw is lodged in the distal-dorsal triquetrum and directed toward the distal-volar portion of the capitate. In this way each screw skips the other in a given bone. Arthroscopy can be very helpful to ascertain the correct position of the critical capitolunate guidewire (**Fig. 10**).

The wires are slightly backed out and cancellous bone graft (harvested from the distal radius) is now inserted. An opened needle cap, working as a cannula, and the scope trocar, working as a plunger, is an inexpensive system for delivery of the bone graft inside the joint (**Fig. 11**).

Once the bone-grafting step is completed, the midcarpal joint is again reduced, and the guidewires reinserted in their previous position. A fluoroscopic assessment is recommended. The appropriate-length screw is now inserted after drilling its canal in the usual fashion. The radiolunate K-wire is removed at this stage. The portals are closed with paper tape except for the scaphoid portal, where an intradermal stitch is used. Protected range of motion is commenced at about 2 weeks (**Fig. 12**).

SUMMARY

Wrist arthroscopy can be performed without infusing fluid, as simple traction will suffice to maintain the working space. The lack of tissue infiltration by fluid keeps soft tissues in pristine condition if open surgery is needed after the arthroscopic exploration. The fact that the dry technique makes fluid distension irrelevant opens a new set of possibilities by combining arthroscopy with moderate-sized incisions (**Fig. 13**). Although in truth any modification of a technique with which one is familiar can be regarded with major reticence, the advantages of the dry technique merit giving it a try. Any accomplished wrist arthroscopist will have minimal problems in swapping from the wet to the dry, and vice versa.

REFERENCES

1. del Piñal F, García-Bernal FJ, Pisani D, et al. Dry arthroscopy of the wrist: surgical technique. J Hand Surg Am 2007;32:119–23.
2. Doi K, Hattori Y, Otsuka K, et al. Intra-articular fractures of the distal aspect of the radius: arthroscopically assisted reduction compared with open reduction and internal fixation. J Bone Joint Surg Am 1999;81:1093–110.
3. Ruch DS, Vallee J, Poehling GG, et al. Arthroscopic reduction versus fluoroscopic reduction in the

management of intra-articular distal radius fractures. Arthroscopy 2004;20:225–30.

4. Varitimidis SE, Basdekis GK, Dailiana ZH, et al. Treatment of intra-articular fractures of the distal radius: fluoroscopic or arthroscopic reduction? J Bone Joint Surg Br 2008;90:778–85.

5. del Pinal F, Garcia-Bernal FG, Studer A, et al. Explosion type articular distal radius fractures: technique and results of volar locking plate under dry arthroscopy guidance. Presented at the FESSH Meeting in Poznan. Poland, 2009. [Book of abstracts: A0180].

6. del Piñal F. Dry arthroscopy of the wrist: its role in the management of articular distal radius fractures. Scand J Surg 2008;97:298–304.

7. del Piñal F. Treatment of explosion-type distal radius fractures. In: del Piñal F, Mathoulin C, Luchetti C, editors. Arthroscopic management of distal radius fractures. Berlin: Springer Verlag; 2010. p. 41–65.

8. del Piñal F, García-Bernal FJ, Delgado J, et al. Correction of malunited intra-articular distal radius fractures with an inside-out osteotomy technique. J Hand Surg Am 2006;31:1029–34.

9. Edwards CC III, Harasztic J, McGillivary GR, et al. Intra-articular distal radius fractures: arthroscopic assessment of radiographically assisted reduction. J Hand Surg Am 2001;26:1036–41.

10. Lutsky K, Boyer MI, Steffen JA, et al. Arthroscopic assessment of intra-articular distal radius fractures after open reduction and internal fixation from a volar approach. J Hand Surg Am 2008;33:476–84.

11. del Piñal F. Arthroscopic-assisted osteotomy for intraarticular malunion of the distal radius. In: del Piñal F, Mathoulin C, Luchetti C, editors. Arthroscopic management of distal radius fractures. Berlin: Springer Verlag; 2010. p. 191–209.

12. del Piñal F, Cagigal L, García-Bernal FJ, et al. Arthroscopically guided osteotomy for management of intra-articular distal radius malunions. J Hand Surg Am 2010;35:392–7.

13. Ho PC. Arthroscopic partial wrist fusion. Tech Hand Up Extrem Surg 2008;12:242–65.

Arthroscopic Hemiresection for Stage II-III Trapeziometacarpal Osteoarthritis

Joshua M. Abzug, MD[a,*], A. Lee Osterman, MD[b,c]

KEYWORDS

- Hemitrapeziectomy • Carpometacarpal arthroscopy
- Trapeziometacarpal arthritis • Basal joint

The thumb trapeziometacarpal joint, otherwise known as the first carpometacarpal (CMC) joint or basal joint of the thumb, experiences significant loading throughout many routine activities. Therefore, degenerative arthritis of this joint is quite common, with age-adjusted radiographic evidence of arthritis present in 15% of females and 7% of males.[1] In addition, one-third of postmenopausal women have been shown to have arthritic changes present.[2]

The anatomy of the trapeziometacarpal joint is quite complex, due to the ligamentous structures present that enable the joint to have motion in multiple planes including abduction/adduction, flexion/extension, and axial rotation. The initial description of the ligamentous anatomy was in 1742 by Weitbrecht, in his book entitled *Syndesmology*.[3] Subsequently, the ligamentous anatomy has been further elucidated and currently 16 ligamentous structures are known to provide stability to the trapeziometacarpal joint, trapezium and second metacarpal, and scaphotrapezial-trapezoid joint. These ligaments have been shown by Bettinger and colleagues[4] to function as a tension band to prevent instability from cantilever bending forces. The forces placed on the trapeziometacarpal joint occur during pinch as loads are transferred to the trapezium because of a lack of base support from the mobile scaphoid.

Multiple ligaments have been proposed as the most important ligament in preventing trapeziometacarpal subluxation. Van Brenk and colleagues[5] suggested that the dorsoradial collateral ligament was most important by serially sectioning the capsular ligaments. Zancolli and Cozzi[6] have proposed that aberrant slips of the abductor pollicis longus place excessive compressive forces on the dorsoradial aspect of the joint, thus leading to subluxation and arthrosis. Pelligrini[7] has popularized the theory that the volar beak ligament undergoes attritional changes, possibly due to estrogen-type hormones, thus leading to dorsal subluxation of the joint.

HISTORY TAKING AND PHYSICAL EXAMINATION

Patients most commonly present with a chief complaint of pain in the region of the base of their thumb. The pain can be localized to either the

The authors have nothing to disclose.

[a] Department of Orthopaedic Surgery, University of Maryland School of Medicine, 22 South Greene Street, Suite S11B, Baltimore, MD 21201, USA

[b] Department of Orthopaedic Surgery, The Philadelphia Hand Center, Thomas Jefferson University Hospital, 834 Chestnut Street, Suite G114, Philadelphia, PA 19107, USA

[c] The Philadelphia Hand Center, 700 South Henderson Road, Suite 200, King of Prussia, PA 19406, USA

* Corresponding author. Department of Orthopaedic Surgery, University of Maryland School of Medicine, 22 South Greene Street, Suite S11B, Baltimore, Maryland, MD 21201.

E-mail address: jabzug1@yahoo.com

hand.theclinics.com

dorsal aspect or the volar, thenar eminence. Symptoms often are attributable to pinching and gripping activities, such as turning keys, opening doorknobs, or opening jar tops.

Physical examination can identify tenderness to palpation about the trapeziometacarpal joint, and a positive grind test may be present. Other conditions in the differential diagnosis should be ruled out, including de Quervain tenosynovitis, scapho-trapeziotrapezoid (STT) arthritis, and scaphoid pathology. In addition, carpal tunnel syndrome and trigger thumb/fingers are commonly present in the population with trapeziometacarpal arthritis, and therefore the etiology of the patient's complaints must be elucidated.

RADIOGRAPHIC CLASSIFICATION

The most commonly used staging system for trapeziometacarpal arthritis is that of Eaton and Littler from their classic 1973 article. Stage I is the synovitis phase, which occurs prior to the development of significant capsular laxity. The radiograph may show mild widening of the joint space due to the presence of an effusion; however, the articular surfaces are congruent and no more than one-third subluxation of the joint is present in any view. Stage II has significant capsular laxity present with subluxation being at least one-third of the joint. In addition, osteophytes less than 2 mm in diameter are present. In Stage III there is significant joint space narrowing, subchondral sclerosis, and peripheral osteophytes greater than 2 mm in diameter, but a normal STT joint. In Stage IV there is pantrapezial osteoarthritis with narrowing, sclerosis, and osteophytes involving both the trapeziometacarpal and STT joints.[8] There is some blurring of the stages, but they still provide a starting point for a rational treatment plan.

TREATMENT OPTIONS

Early arthritis is typically treated with conservative measures including activity modification, medications, splinting, or injections. Activity modification to avoid pinching, gripping, and twisting may significantly improve a patient's complaints. Nonsteroidal anti-inflammatory drugs are the most commonly used recommended medication, as this class of drugs reduces inflammation, synovitis, and pain. Splinting the trapeziometacarpal joint can decrease pain, reduce mechanical stress, and improve function.[9] Steroid injections into the trapeziometacarpal joint attempt to reduce inflammation and provide pain relief; however, the effects are usually temporary.[10,11]

Surgical treatment is performed when conservative measures fail. Options for Stage II and early Stage III include Eaton ligament reconstruction,[8] Wilson extension osteotomy,[12] arthroscopic debridement with and without biological resurfacing, trapeziectomy with or without ligament reconstruction, prosthetic replacement, and arthrodesis. The remainder of this article focuses on the arthroscopic management of trapeziometacarpal arthritis.

HISTORICAL BACKGROUND

The use of small joint arthroscopy has continued to evolve since the introduction of the Watanabe No. 24 arthroscope in the early 1970s by Yung-Cheng Chen.[13] In 1996, the first clinical article on trapeziometacarpal arthroscopy was published by Menon.[14] This article described the technique of performing an arthroscopic partial trapezium resection and placement of an interpositional arthroplasty. Of the 25 patients presented, three-quarters had complete pain relief. In 1997, Berger[15] published a technique paper illustrating 12 cases of trapeziometacarpal arthroscopy, expanding its use beyond only arthritic conditions. This expansion was further demonstrated in a 1997 article by Osterman and colleagues[16] wherein two groups, one traumatic and one degenerative, both benefited from arthroscopic intervention at the trapeziometacarpal joint.

ARTHROSCOPIC STAGING

The concept of arthroscopic staging of the trapeziometacarpal joint was introduced by Badia in 2006.[17] Stage I is characterized by diffuse synovitis without significant cartilage loss, and frequently ligamentous laxity of the volar capsule is present. This stage is not usually encountered as patients are typically more advanced when surgical intervention is undertaken. However, if it is present simple synovectomy with or without electrothermal shrinkage, based on ligamentous laxity, is the preferred treatment. Stage II is present when there is focal wear of the central to dorsal articular surface of the trapezium. Classically this is the indication for osteotomy of the metacarpal base, in order to place the thumb in a more extended and abducted position to alter the vector forces across the trapeziometacarpal joint. However, this stage can also be treated with arthroscopic interventions, as described later in this article. Stage III has diffuse articular cartilage loss on the trapezium with or without metacarpal base articular cartilage loss. This stage is also amenable to treatment with arthroscopic hemiresection of the trapezium.

SURGICAL TECHNIQUE
Diagnostic Arthroscopy

Anesthesia is provided to the patient with either general anesthesia or regional anesthesia with sedation. The patient is then placed supine on the operating room table and a nonsterile tourniquet is applied, set to 250 mm Hg. After the affected extremity is prepped and draped in a usual fashion, the standard wrist arthroscopy tower is assembled. A single Chinese finger trap is placed on the thumb, and the forearm is adequately padded as it is placed against the traction tower. The thumb finger trap is placed in the traction tower and a sterile elastic bandage (Coban; 3M, St Paul, MN, USA) is used to secure the forearm, wrist, and hand to the traction tower, while leaving the thumb and trapeziometacarpal joint free. Traction is set between 5 and 10 pounds (2.7–4.5 kg) (**Fig. 1**).

The next step is to locate the trapeziometacarpal joint by moving the thumb passively and palpating the metacarpal proximally until a depression is felt. At this level, the abductor pollicis longus and extensor pollicis brevis tendons should be easily palpated and marked. A hemostat is then used to mark the 1-R portal, which is directly radial to the abductor pollicis longus tendon at the level of the trapeziometacarpal joint. The 1-U portal, directly ulnar to the extensor pollicis brevis tendon at the level of the joint, is also marked. There usually is approximately 1 cm between these portals (**Fig. 2**).

Once the setup is complete, the tourniquet is inflated and saline is injected into the trapeziometacarpal joint to distend it. Either portal can be used for injection; however, it is imperative to note the angulation required to enter the joint. Subsequently, a number 11 scalpel is used to incise the skin only at the marking for the 1-R portal. A blunt

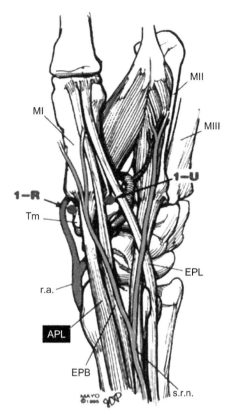

Fig. 2. Underlying anatomy in relation to trapeziometacarpal arthroscopic portals. APL, abductor pollicis longus; EPB, extensor pollicis brevis; EPL, extensor pollicis longus; MI, metacarpal I; MII, metacarpal II; MIII, metacarpal III; r.a, radial artery; s.r.n., superficial radial nerve; Tm, trapezium; 1-R, 1-radial; 1-U, 1-ulnar.

hemostat is then used to gently spread down to the trapeziometacarpal joint capsule. Blunt dissection is mandatory to minimize potential injury to the dorsal radial sensory nerve branches, the radial artery, and the aforementioned tendons. The hemostat is now used to puncture through the joint capsule. Confirmation of entering the joint is present when the surgeon visualizes the egress of the previously injected saline.

The arthroscope is now introduced into the trapeziometacarpal joint (**Fig. 3**). One can use a 1.5-mm, 1.9-mm, or 2.7-mm arthroscope, based on preference. Attention is now turned to the 1-U portal, which is established by placing an 18-gauge needle into the joint and then following the same steps previously mentioned to establish the 1-R portal (**Fig. 4**). Visualization initially can be limited, due to the arthritic condition, and therefore the joint may have to be debrided to allow for adequate inspection.

The synovium is removed by using a 2.0-mm arthroscopic full-radius shaver attached to

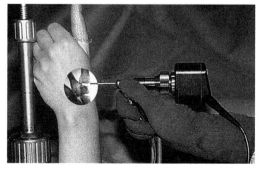

Fig. 1. Trapeziometacarpal arthroscopic setup and equipment, including a 1.9-mm 30° short-barrel arthroscope, 2.0-mm shaving instruments, a short probe, an 18-gauge hypodermic needle, and thermal shrinking probes.

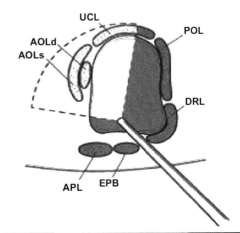

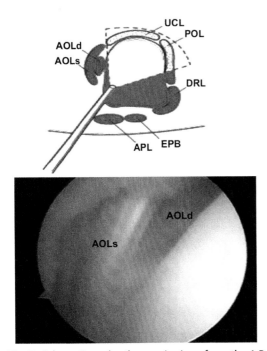

Fig. 3. Schematic and arthroscopic views from the 1-R portal. AOLd, anterior oblique ligament deep; AOLs, anterior oblique ligament superficial; APL, abductor pollicis longus; DRL, dorsoradial ligament; EPB, extensor pollicis brevis; POL, posterior oblique ligament; UCL, ulnar collateral ligament.

suction. Once visualization is adequate, the entire trapeziometacarpal joint should be systematically inspected. The authors prefer to begin the inspection by evaluating the base of the first metacarpal. This landmark is easy to identify, as confirmation can be obtained simply by moving the thumb and visualizing intra-articular movement of the base of the metacarpal. Following this, attention is turned to the trapezium where its entire surface is visualized from ulnar to radial to evaluate for cartilaginous defects and eburnated bone. While working volarly, one can inspect the oblique ligament and assess its integrity using a probe. The dorsoradial ligament can also be visualized on the dorsoradial side of the joint. Once the entire joint has been assessed, an arthroscopic stage is assigned based on the aforementioned classification.

Hemitrapeziectomy

If the patient is arthroscopic Stage II or III, then hemitrapeziectomy is performed by using a full-radius shaver to remove the articular cartilage present on the distal surface of the trapezium. The authors have found this to be is more efficient than a burr, as the burr is better suited for removing bone than cartilage. Once the cartilage

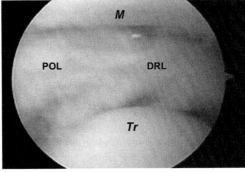

Fig. 4. Schematic and arthroscopic views from the 1-U portal. AOLs, anterior oblique ligament superficial; AOLd, anterior oblique ligament deep; APL, abductor pollicis longus; DRL, dorsoradial ligament; EPB, extensor pollicis brevis; M, metacarpal; POL, posterior oblique ligament; Tr, trapezium; UCL, ulnar collateral ligament.

has been removed, a full-radius round burr is introduced through one of the portals and under fluoroscopic guidance the distal half of the trapezium is removed. The authors have found it easiest to work with the burr in the 1-R portal and then sweep the burr from ulnar to radial to contour a smooth, flat surface. It is imperative to remove any osteophytes that may be present between the trapezium and base of the second metacarpal. The joint should intermittently be irrigated and suctioned to remove any debris/loose bodies as well as to cool the burr. Adequate resection is confirmed with fluoroscopy (**Fig. 5**).

Stability Assessment and Treatment

Once the hemitrapeziectomy is completed, joint stability should be assessed. If there is laxity present, thermal capsulodesis can be performed to stabilize the joint. A 0.045-inch (1.143 mm) Kirschner wire can be added for additional stability by ensuring joint reduction and placing the pin from the first metacarpal to the residual trapezium or

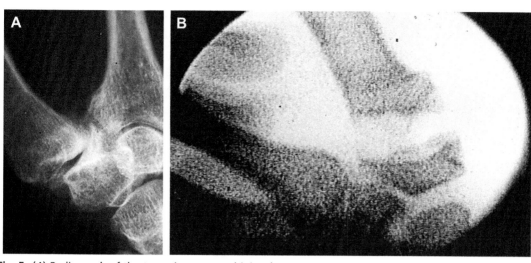

Fig. 5. (*A*) Radiograph of the trapeziometacarpal joint demonstrating Stage II osteoarthritis. (*B*) Intraoperative fluoroscopic imaging confirming 2 to 4 mm of trapezial resection. Note the lack of osteophyte between the first and second metacarpal bases.

scaphoid. Slight abduction of the first metacarpal is recommended to prevent proximal migration.[9]

An alternative to placing the Kirschner wire is to perform a suspensionplasty using a suture button technique.[18] The Mini-TightRope (Arthrex, Naples, FL, USA) is inserted from the first metacarpal base to the second metacarpal base to prevent subsidence of the newly created trapeziometacarpal space. The technique is performed by making a skin incision on the radial aspect of the first metacarpal base, just volar to the abductor pollicis longus tendon. Blunt dissection is performed with a hemostat down to bone. A 1.2-mm guide wire is then placed from the volar-radial first metacarpal base to the dorsal-ulnar aspect of the second metacarpal base. Cox and colleagues[18] stated that the orientation should be oblique in nature, slightly distal on the second metacarpal, to provide a better vector of tension to prevent subsidence. Accurate placement of the guide wire is confirmed with fluoroscopy.

Once the guide wire is palpable between the second and third metacarpals, a small skin incision is made and blunt dissection with a hemostat is performed to visualize the ulnar part of the second metacarpal where the guide wire is exiting. The next step is to overdrill the guide wire through all 4 cortices with a 2.7-mm cannulated drill. The guide wire should be maintained after the overdrilling, to allow for passage of the cannulated passer that clears debris for placement of the Mini-TightRope. Subsequently, the guide wire is removed and the oblong button of the Mini-TightRope is passed through the cannulated passer from ulnar to radial, to exit at the base of the thumb metacarpal. Once passed, the passer

is removed and the oblong button is placed flush against the volar-radial aspect of the thumb metacarpal without any interposing soft tissue.

Attention is now turned to the round button, which is similarly placed directly against the ulnar border of the second metacarpal without any interposing soft tissue. A provisional knot that removes all slack is now placed to assess tension. Fluoroscopy is used to ensure adequate suspension and under live image a ballottement test is performed to demonstrate a lack of subsidence (**Fig. 6**). In addition, it is important to ensure overtensioning has not occurred resulting in impingement between the first and second metacarpal bases.

Once the surgeon is satisfied with the tension, additional knots are placed and the suture ends are cut. The wounds are closed in a standard manner.

Interposition

Placement of interposition into the hemitrapeziectomy space is done according to the surgeon's preference. Various options exist including autograft, allograft, or prosthetic material. Autograft options include the flexor carpi radialis or palmaris longus tendons. Fascia lata allograft has also been used. Prosthetic options include Artelon spacer (Artimplant, Vastra Frolunda, Sweden) or Graftjacket (Wright Medical Technology, Inc., Arlington, TN, USA). Graftjacket is an acellular dermal matrix allograft manufactured to be approximately 1 mm thick. After it is rehydrated in normal saline for 10 to 15 minutes, it can be folded to double its thickness and cut to an appropriate size for placement in the newly created space. The Artelon spacer, composed of a polycaprolactone-based polyurethane urea that

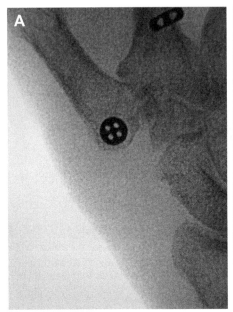
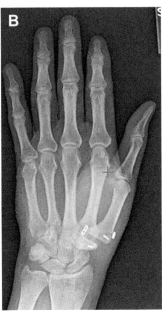

Fig. 6. (*A*) Intraoperative fluoroscopic image of the Mini-TightRope in place between the bases of the first and second metacarpals. (*B*) Radiograph demonstrating placement of the Mini-TightRope between the first and second metacarpal bases.

hydrolyzes over several years and allows native cell incorporation, is the authors' preferred technique. It is cut to the appropriate size and placed into the newly formed space through the 1-R portal.

After placement of an interposition, the portals are closed with simple nylon sutures and the patient is placed in a thumb spica splint.

Aftercare

Patients are placed in a plaster thumb spica splint for 2 weeks regardless of the procedure performed. At the 2-week postoperative visit, the splint and sutures are removed. If a Kirschner wire had been placed for added stability, a custom thermoplast splint is fabricated and worn for an additional 2 weeks at which time the pin is removed and range-of-motion exercises are begun. By contrast, if a suspensionplasty is performed with the Mini-TightRope, early range-of-motion exercises are begun at the 2-week postoperative visit.

OUTCOMES

Until recently only results of short-term follow-up had been reported regarding the role of trapeziometacarpal arthroscopy. However, over the last few years multiple articles have demonstrated the successful use of this technique over a longer time period.

In 2008, Earp and colleagues[19] presented their results of 15 procedures in 14 patients treated with an arthroscopic hemitrapeziectomy and

tendon interposition. At approximately 1 year of follow-up average pain scores decreased from 8.6 points preoperatively to 1.8 points postoperatively. The overwhelming majority of patients reported that they felt much better, with the remainder reporting that they felt somewhat better. At the most recent follow-up grip strength had returned to more than 90% of the contralateral side, tip pinch strength was 90% of the contralateral side, and lateral pinch strength was 85% of the contralateral side.

Also in 2008, Adams and colleagues[20] reported their results of 17 patients using arthroscopic hemitrapeziectomy and placement of Graftjacket as interposition. After an average of 17 months, all patients reported symptomatic relief and 88% reported no, or only occasional, pain with activity. Average grip strength was 18.5 kg and average pinch strength was 3.9 kg. All patients who worked were able to return to their occupation postoperatively. The only complication noted was one case of postoperative ulnar neuropathy in a patient who underwent an axillary nerve block for anesthesia.

In 2009, Hofmeister and colleagues[21] presented the longest-term follow-up result of patients undergoing arthroscopic hemitrapeziectomy. Their study had an average follow-up of 7.6 years (range 6.5–8.4 years) involving 18 patients. Significant improvement in a "thumb function score" was present, with scores improving from 60 to 90. Three patients were noted to have a mildly positive grind test and one patient had asymptomatic laxity

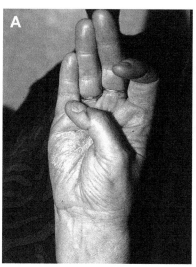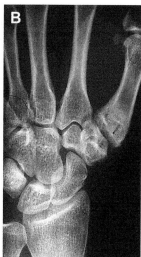

Fig. 7. (A, B) 7.5-year follow-up after interposition arthroplasty. Note alignment and preservation of trapeziometacarpal space.

of the trapeziometacarpal joint. All patients could oppose the thumb to the small finger; however, composite range of motion of the thumb axis decreased by 20%. Statistically significant improvements were present in key pinch strength and tip pinch strength. Radiographic evaluation at long-term follow-up compared with the immediate postoperative period demonstrated 1.8 mm (range 0–4 mm) of metacarpal subsidence (**Fig. 7**).

Four complications were noted including two cases of dorsal radial nerve neuritis, one of which was still present at the latest follow-up. In addition, there was one patient who had a prolonged hematoma with overlying skin necrosis that went on to resolve, and one patient with a flexor pollicis longus rupture that occurred 6 weeks postoperatively who was treated with primary repair.[21]

In 2010, Edwards and Ramsey[22] published the only prospective study to evaluate arthroscopic hemitrapeziectomy. Twenty-three patients with Eaton Stage III trapeziometacarpal arthritis underwent arthroscopic hemitrapeziectomy and thermal capsular modification without interposition. These patients were followed prospectively for a minimum of 4 years. Preoperatively the average Disabilities of the Arm, Shoulder, and Hand (DASH) score was 61 (range 45–69) whereas at the 3-month postoperative visit the DASH had improved to 10 (range 7–12). This improvement was maintained over the 4-year period: CMC palpation and grind tests, DASH scores, pain scores, grip and pinch strengths, motion, and patient satisfaction remained unchanged.

In addition, average analog pain scores significantly improved from 8.3 (range 6–10) preoperatively to 1.5 (range 0–2) at 3 months postoperatively

and 1.1 (range 0–2) at 4 years postoperatively. First metacarpal subsidence was found to be 3 mm (range 2–4) at the 3-month postoperative visit, and this remained the same at the 4-year postoperative visit. The only complication noted was a painful neuroma that developed secondary to pin placement.[22]

SUMMARY

Trapeziometacarpal osteoarthritis is an extremely common problem, due to the anatomy of the first ray and the forces applied to the trapeziometacarpal joint throughout activities of daily living. Numerous treatment options exist, and continue to be developed, for this problem. The current goal is to eliminate pain and restore function and strength in a timely manner. As technology continues to improve, new advances allow for earlier return to function with minimally invasive techniques. Arthroscopic hemitrapeziectomy combined with interposition arthroplasty and/or suspensionplasty is a treatment option for Stage II and III trapeziometacarpal arthritis that uses a minimally invasive technique and allows for earlier return of function. Recent long-term follow-up studies have demonstrated the significant improvements over prolonged periods.

REFERENCES

1. Haara MM, Heliovaara M, Kroger H, et al. Osteoarthritis in the carpometacarpal joint of the thumb: prevalence and associations with disability and mortality. J Bone Joint Surg Am 2004;86:1452–7.

2. Armstrong AL, Hunter JB, Davis TR. The prevalence of degenerative arthritis of the base of the thumb in postmenopausal women. J Hand Surg Br 1994;19: 340–1.

3. Weitbrecht J. Syndesmology. Philadelphia: WB Saunders; 1969 [originally published 1742].

4. Bettinger PC, Linscheid RL, Berger RA, et al. An anatomic study of the stabilizing ligaments of the trapezium and trapeziometacarpal joint. J Hand Surg Am 1999;24A:786–98.

5. Van Brenk B, Richards RR, Mackay MB, et al. A biomechanical assessment of ligaments preventing dorsoradial subluxation of the trapeziometacarpal joint. J Hand Surg Am 1998;23:607–11.

6. Zancolli EA, Cozzi EP. The trapeziometacarpal joint: anatomy and mechanics. In: Zancolli E, Cozzi EP, editors. Atlas of surgical anatomy of the hand. New York: Churchill Livingstone; 1992. p. 443–4.

7. Pelligrini VD. Pathomechanics of the thumb trapeziometacarpal joint. Hand Clin (Thumb Arthritis) 2001; 17:151–68.

8. Eaton RG, Littler JW. Ligament reconstruction for the painful thumb carpometacarpal joint. J Bone Joint Surg Am 1973;55:1655–66.

9. Yao J, Park MJ. Early treatment of degenerative arthritis of the thumb carpometacarpal joint. Hand Clin 2008;24:251–61.

10. Joshi R. Intra-articular corticosteroid injection for first carpometacarpal osteoarthritis. J Rheumatol 2005; 32:1305–6.

11. Meenagh GK, Patton J, Kynes C, et al. A randomized controlled trial of intra-articular corticosteroid injection of the carpometacarpal joint of the thumb in osteoarthritis. Ann Rheum Dis 2004;63:1260–3.

12. Parker WL, Linscheid RL, Amadio PC. Long-term outcomes of first metacarpal extension osteotomy in the treatment of carpal-metacarpal osteoarthritis. J Hand Surg Am 2008;33:1737–43.

13. Chen YC. Arthroscopy of the wrist and finger joints. Orthop Clin North Am 1979;10:723–33.

14. Menon J. Arthroscopic management of trapeziometacarpal arthritis of the thumb. Arthroscopy 1996;12: 581–7.

15. Berger RA. Technique for arthroscopic evaluation of the first carpometacarpal joint. J Hand Surg Am 1997;22:1077–80.

16. Osterman AL, Culp R, Bednar J. Arthroscopy of the thumb carpometacarpal joint. Arthroscopy 1997; 13:411.

17. Badia A. Trapeziometacarpal arthroscopy: a classification and treatment algorithm. Hand Clin 2006;22: 153–63.

18. Cox CA, Zlotolow DA, Yao J. Suture button suspensionplasty after arthroscopic hemitrapeziectomy for treatment of thumb carpometacarpal arthritis. Arthroscopy 2010;26:1395–403.

19. Earp BE, Leung AC, Blazar PE, et al. Arthroscopic hemitrapeziectomy with tendon interposition for arthritis at the first carpometacarpal joint. Tech Hand Up Extrem Surg 2008;12:38–42.

20. Adams JE, Merten SM, Steinmann SP. Arthroscopic interposition arthroplasty of the first carpometacarpal joint. J Hand Surg Eur Vol 2008;32:268–74.

21. Hofmeister EP, Leak RS, Culp RW, et al. Arthroscopic hemitrapeziectomy for first carpometacarpal arthritis: results at 7-year follow-up. Hand (N Y) 2009;4:24–8.

22. Edwards SG, Ramsey PN. Prospective outcomes of stage-III thumb carpometacarpal arthritis treated with arthroscopic hemitrapeziectomy and thermal capsular modification without interposition. J Hand Surg Am 2010;35:566–71.

Bone-Preserving Arthroscopic Options For Treatment of Thumb Basilar Joint Arthritis

Julie E. Adams, MD[a,*], Scott P. Steinmann, MD[b],
Randall W. Culp, MD[c]

KEYWORDS

- Arthroscopy • Bone preservation • Basilar joint arthritis
- Trapezium • CMC joint arthritis
- Trapeziometacarpal arthritis

While trapeziectomy with or without interposition arthroplasty and ligament reconstruction or suspensionplasty has been demonstrated to have a high rate of satisfactory outcomes, recent interest has focused on arthroscopy because of its perceived limited invasive nature as well as its versatility. In addition, using the arthroscope other options are available that preserve all or part of the trapezium in order to limit subsidence of the thumb axis, preserve grip and pinch strength, and retain later options for joint reconstruction, should that become necessary.[1–9]

OPTIONS IN ARTHROSCOPIC MANAGEMENT

Arthroscopy may be useful as a staging or diagnostic procedure as well as a therapeutic one.[2,8,10–12] Options include arthroscopic visualization of the extent of joint changes, with simple debridement or synovectomy or capsular shrinkage of ligaments, debridement of arthritis, and hemitrapeziectomy with or without interposition arthroplasty. In addition, assessment of the cartilage may be performed, with an intraoperative decision being made for further interventions, for example, conversion to an open procedure such as a metacarpal osteotomy, an open joint reconstruction such as hemitrapeziectomy or complete trapeziectomy, and/or ligament reconstruction.

In patients for whom arthroscopy reveals minimal joint changes and in whom the articular surface is mostly intact, one can consider synovial debridement and capsular shrinkage with a heat probe. However, those with more extensive changes, such as full-thickness cartilage loss or frank osteophyte formation, may require a joint resurfacing procedure such as arthroscopic or open debridement, or hemitrapeziectomy or complete trapeziectomy with or without interposition arthroplasty. In cases of partial loss of the volar cartilage and attenuation of the anterior oblique ligament, patients may be considered for an extension osteotomy or a resurfacing procedure.[2,3,10,12]

SURGICAL TECHNIQUE

The surgical technique begins by suspending the thumb from a traction tower with 5 to 8 lb (2.3–3.6 kg) of traction.[1,13,14] Following suspension of the thumb in the traction tower, surface landmarks

[a] Department of Orthopaedic Surgery, University of Minnesota, 2450 Riverside Avenue R 200, Minneapolis, MN 55454, USA
[b] Department of Orthopaedic Surgery, Mayo Clinic, 200 First Street South West, Rochester, MN 55905, USA
[c] Thomas Jefferson University, The Philadelphia Hand Center, 700 South Henderson Road, King of Prussia, PA 19406, USA
* Corresponding author.
E-mail address: adams854@umn.edu

Hand Clin 27 (2011) 355–359
doi:10.1016/j.hcl.2011.05.005
0749-0712/11/$ – see front matter © 2011 Elsevier Inc. All rights reserved.

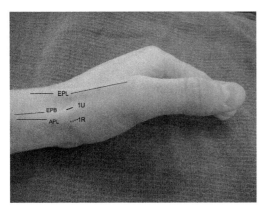

Fig. 1. Landmarks and portal sites. Portals: 1-U, 2-R. Landmarks: APL, abductor pollicis longus; EPB, extensor pollicis longus; EPL, extensor pollicis longus.

are marked (**Fig. 1**). The 1-R (radial) and 1-U (ulnar) portals (**Fig. 2**) are used, and either may be designated the starting portal. The 1-R portal is created at the trapeziometacarpal joint between the abductor pollicus longus (APL) and the flexor carpi radialis (FCR) tendons. The closer this portal is made toward the FCR, the better the triangulation and visualization becomes. This portal is useful to visualize the dorsal radial ligament, the palmar oblique ligament, and the thumb ulnar collateral ligament of the carpometacarpal (CMC) joint, as well as the intermetacarpal ligament and the insertion of the anterior oblique ligament. The 1-U portal is adjacent to the extensor pollicus brevis (EPB) tendon on the ulnar side, and this portal site is closer to branches of the superficial radial nerve as well as the radial artery. To avoid injury to these structures, it is best to establish portals in the standard fashion in which the skin is only incised and a small hemostat is used to bluntly dissect down to the capsule. This portal does enter through the dorsal radial ligament, or between it and the palmar oblique ligament, and allows for visualization of the anterior oblique ligament.[1,2]

Following marking of the landmarks and intended portal sites, a small-gauge needle is used to enter the intended portal site and insufflate the joint with saline. Because of the small spaces involved, it is possible to inadvertently enter the scaphotrapezo-trapezoidal joint, so a mini-fluoroscopy unit is useful to confirm appropriate portal placement before starting the procedure. The portals are made in standard fashion as already noted, with blunt dissection and care taken to avoid injury to subcutaneous structures.

A second accessory dorsal-distal (D-2) portal has been described by Slutsky[4] for improved visualization of the medial aspect of the trapezium, and is located 1 cm distal to the cleft between the

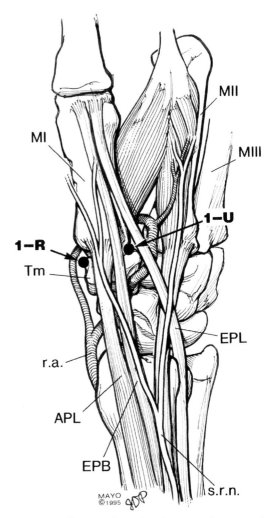

Fig. 2. Line drawing depicting the 1-R and 1-U portals and landmarks. APL, abductor pollicis longus; EPB, extensor pollicis longus; EPL, extensor pollicis longus; MI, first metacarpal; MII, second metacarpal; MIII, third metacarpal; r.a., radial artery; s.r.n., superficial radial nerve; Tm, trapezium. (*From* Berger RA. A technique for arthroscopic evaluation of the first carpometacarpal joint. J Hand Surg Am 1997;22:1077–80.)

junction of the bases of the index and thumb metacarpals just ulnar to the extensor pollicis longus tendon. The portal site is made with care taken to avoid the radial artery, and a 22-gauge needle is inserted in a proximal-radial and palmar direction.

A 1.9-mm arthroscope may be used, or a slightly larger one such as the 2.3- or 2.7-mm wrist arthroscope. Initially the procedure may be difficult, given the small joint space, but with further work the joint space is enlarged and visualization becomes easier. Diagnostic arthroscopy is performed to evaluate the extent of bony and cartilage changes as well as the capsular changes. A radiofrequency ablator or cautery is helpful in removing soft tissue and performing capsular shrinkage if laxity is present. The small joint shaver, on the order of 2.9 to 3.5 mm, and a burr may be used as well. Following completion of the diagnostic arthroscopy, attention is then turned to synovectomy and soft-tissue debridement, with or without capsular shrinkage.

If the cartilage surface is poor, one can consider bony debridement and an interposition arthroplasty. Studies of open complete trapeziectomy have suggested that resection of the arthritic surface alone without interposition may be adequate for pain relief, although many surgeons continue to place an interposition material.[5–7,15–19]

No comparative studies between interposition and no interposition have been performed following arthroscopy; however, one series suggests that arthroscopic debridement alone may be satisfactory, and that interposition may not be necessary.[11]

A 2.9- to 3.5-mm burr is useful for removal of the distal portion of the trapezium down to subchondral bone; 2 to 4 mm of bone may be removed. This method can be assessed easily by taking into account the diameter of the burr as a measuring device intraoperatively. It is essential to remove the bony osteophytes beneath the volar ulnar edge of the second metacarpal, thus avoiding that it continues to be a source of pain. After the initial work is done, burring may be continued under fluoroscopy to ensure that adequate bone has been removed. Placement of the interposition material, if desired, may be performed following this action.

A variety of materials have been used, including autologous tissue or allogeneic tissue as well as manufactured or processed materials.[8,11,20,21] Limited data are available regarding outcomes following such procedures; however, recent series suggest that it has a satisfactory rate of good to excellent outcomes. Such interposition materials may include autologous palmaris longus, part of the FCR, gelfoam, GraftJacket (Wright Medical Technology, Arlington, TN, USA), and Artelon (Small Bone Innovations, Morrisville, PA, USA), among others.[3,8–10,13,14]

The interposition material, if used, is inserted and traction let off the thumb gradually to secure the interposition material between the base of the metacarpus and the remaining trapezium. The interposition material is passed through the joint through a portal by use of a small hemostat. A second hemostat may be used to pull the material from the other portal site. The portals are then closed, and a thumb spica splint applied. Immobilization is continued for a period of 6 weeks, and routine postoperative radiographs are obtained at follow-up (**Figs. 3** and **4**).

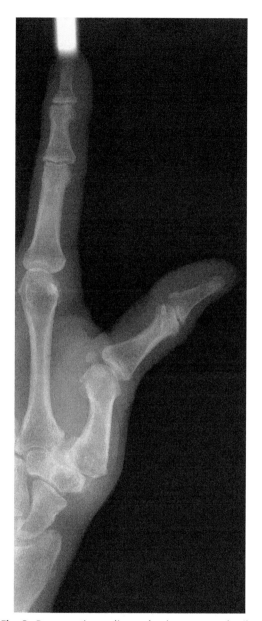

Fig. 3. Preoperative radiographs demonstrate basilar joint arthritis of the thumb.

OUTCOMES

Although this procedure is relatively new, increasing information is becoming available regarding outcomes following arthroscopic treatment of thumb CMC joint arthritis.

In one study of 17 thumbs with symptomatic laxity of the basilar joint of the thumb, patients underwent arthroscopic radiofrequency electrothermal treatment with a monopolar radiofrequency probe. Patients noted improved pain and pinch strength with satisfactory functional status at 2 years' follow-up.[22] In the series described by

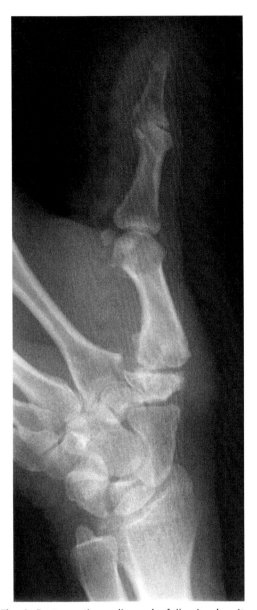

Fig. 4. Postoperative radiographs following hemitrapeziectomy and interposition arthroplasty.

Culp and Rekant,[10] satisfactory outcomes were noted in 88% of 24 patients following joint debridement and shrinkage or partial or complete trapeziectomy.

Hemitrapeziectomy and interposition with a variety of materials has been successful in several series. In one series of 17 patients, outcomes following debridement, hemitrapeziectomy, and interposition arthroplasty with an acellular dermal matrix graft were satisfactory with a mean follow-up of 17 months.[11,21] One of the authors of this article (R.W.C.) has successfully used Artelon as an interposition arthroplasty following arthroscopic debridement in a series of patients. Earp investigated arthroscopic hemitrapeziectomy and tendon interposition arthroplasty with mean follow-up of 11 months, and noted improved pain and a high rate of patient satisfaction.[20] One series of 16 patients with Eaton stages I and II were treated with arthroscopic hemitrapeziectomy with palmaris longus interposition arthroplasty, and were assessed at 12-month follow-up. Results were good to excellent in 75%, but fair in 18% and poor in one patient according to the Mayo score. There were no complications.[21]

A recent series suggests that interposition following hemitrapeziectomy may not be necessary for acceptable results. A series of 23 patients with Eaton stage III basilar joint arthrosis underwent arthroscopic debridement, thermal shrinkage, and hemitrapeziectomy without any interposition, and were followed for longer than 4 years. A high rate of satisfactory outcomes was noted, with 19 of 23 patients endorsing subjective satisfaction. DASH (Disabilities of Arm, Shoulder, and Hand) scores, grip, pinch, motion, and patient satisfaction were preserved from the interval from 3 months to 4 years of follow-up.[11]

Because of the small series and limited use of these techniques, little information is yet available on reconstruction for failures or salvage operations; however, the goal of the procedure is to retain a large portion of the trapezium, making conversion to a complete trapeziectomy a viable option.

In summary, arthroscopic evaluation and treatment of basilar joint arthritis has received recent interest, and recent small series have suggested a satisfactory rate of acceptable outcomes. Further information will likely become available, which will help determine the role of this modality in future treatment of basilar joint arthrosis of the thumb.

In general, arthroscopic assessment and treatment may be used in all Eaton stages of thumb basilar joint arthritis. Early stages (stage 0, I) may be treated with debridement or synovectomy and shrinkage, or consideration of metacarpal osteotomy or ligament reconstruction; later stages (II, III) may be best amenable to debridement and hemitrapeziectomy with or without interposition arthroplasty; and pan-trapezial arthrosis may be treated with a complete trapeziectomy, which may be performed arthroscopically.

REFERENCES

1. Berger RA. A technique for arthroscopic evaluation of the first carpometacarpal joint. J Hand Surg Am 1997;22:1077–80.

2. Badia A. Trapeziometacarpal arthroscopy: a classification and treatment algorithm. Hand Clin 2006;22: 153–63.
3. Adams JE, Steinmann SP, Culp RW. Trapezium-sparing options for thumb carpometacarpal joint arthritis. Am J Orthop (Belle Mead NJ) 2008;37:8–11.
4. Slutsky DJ. The use of a dorsal-distal portal in trapeziometacarpal arthroscopy. Arthroscopy 2007;23: 1244, e1–4.
5. Diao E, Rosenwasser MP, Glickel SZ, et al. Arthritis of the thumb basal joint: old and new treatments for a common condition. Instr Course Lect 2009; 58:551–9.
6. Davis TR, Brady O, Barton NJ, et al. Trapeziectomy alone, with tendon interposition or with ligament reconstruction? J Hand Surg Br 1997;22:689–94.
7. Davis TR, Brady O, Dias JJ. Excision of the trapezium for osteoarthritis of the trapeziometacarpal joint: a study of the benefit of ligament reconstruction or tendon interposition. J Hand Surg Am 2004; 29:1069–77.
8. Badia A. Arthroscopy of the trapeziometacarpal and metacarpophalangeal joints. J Hand Surg Am 2007; 32:707–24.
9. Adams JE, Merten SM, Steinmann SP. Arthroscopic interposition arthroplasty of the first carpometacarpal joint. J Hand Surg Eur Vol 2007;32:268–74.
10. Culp RW, Rekant MS. The role of arthroscopy in evaluating and treating trapeziometacarpal disease. Hand Clin 2001;17:315–9, x–xi.
11. Edwards SG, Ramsey PN. Prospective outcomes of stage III thumb carpometacarpal arthritis treated with arthroscopic hemitrapeziectomy and thermal capsular modification without interposition. J Hand Surg Am 2010;35:566–71.
12. Badia A, Khanchandani P. Treatment of early basal joint arthritis using a combined arthroscopic debridement and metacarpal osteotomy. Tech Hand Up Extrem Surg 2007;11:168–73.
13. Menon J. Arthroscopic management of trapeziometacarpal joint arthritis of the thumb. Arthroscopy 1996;12:581–7.
14. Menon J. Arthroscopic evaluation of the first carpometacarpal joint. J Hand Surg Am 1998;23:757.
15. Jones NF, Maser BM. Treatment of arthritis of the trapeziometacarpal joint with trapeziectomy and hematoma arthroplasty. Hand Clin 2001;17:237–43.
16. Lins RE, Gelberman RH, McKeown L, et al. Basal joint arthritis: trapeziectomy with ligament reconstruction and tendon interposition arthroplasty. J Hand Surg Am 1996;21:202–9.
17. Nylen S, Johnson A, Rosenquist AM. Trapeziectomy and ligament reconstruction for osteoarthrosis of the base of the thumb. A prospective study of 100 operations. J Hand Surg Br 1993;18:616–9.
18. Davis TR, Pace A. Trapeziectomy for trapeziometacarpal joint osteoarthritis: is ligament reconstruction and temporary stabilisation of the pseudarthrosis with a Kirschner wire important? J Hand Surg Eur Vol 2009;34:312–21.
19. Fitzgerald BT, Hofmeister EP. Treatment of advanced carpometacarpal joint disease: trapeziectomy and hematoma arthroplasty. Hand Clin 2008;24:271–6, vi.
20. Earp BE, Leung AC, Blazar PE, et al. Arthroscopic hemitrapeziectomy with tendon interposition for arthritis at the first carpometacarpal joint. Tech Hand Up Extrem Surg 2008;12:38–42.
21. Pegoli L, Parolo C, Ogawa T, et al. Arthroscopic evaluation and treatment by tendon interpositional arthroplasty of first carpometacarpal joint arthritis. Hand Surg 2007;12:35–9.
22. Chu PJ, Lee HM, Chung LJ, et al. Electrothermal treatment of thumb basal joint instability. Arthroscopy 2009;25:290–5.

Arthroscopic Reduction and Percutaneous Fixation of Fifth Carpometacarpal Fracture Dislocations

David J. Slutsky, MD[a,b,*]

KEYWORDS

- Arthroscopy • Fifth carpometacarpal joint
- Anatomic reduction • Volar articular fragment

RATIONALE

Arthroscopy of the first carpometacarpal (CMC) joint has become routine. The literature contains multiple reports of arthroscopic-guided reduction and percutaneous pin fixation of Bennett fractures involving the first carpometacarpal joint. The same techniques can be applied to fracture dislocations involving the fifth CMC joint. This situation is one whereby arthroscopy is definitely of benefit, because the articular fracture fragment is often volar, and difficult to visualize and reduce from a dorsal approach.

ANATOMY AND PATHOMECHANICS

Nakamura and colleagues[1] studied 80 cadaver arms and described the CMC joint in detail. Two distinct dorsal ligaments were identified that attached to the dorsal aspect of the fifth metacarpal (MC). One of these extended from the ulnar base of the fifth MC to the hamate (fifth MC ulnar-side base–hamate ligament) and the other from the radial base of the fifth metacarpal to the hamate, and sometimes to the fourth metacarpal ulnar base (fourth MC ulnar-side base–fifth MC radial-side base ligament). There was an intermetacarpal ligament that attached the radial base of the fifth metacarpal to the ulnar base of the fourth metacarpal. There was one volar ligament that attached to the fifth MC base and extended either to the hook of the hamate or to the ulnar base of the fourth MC. There were no intra-articular ligaments except for one, located between the third/fourth MC and the capitate/hamate.

Dzwierzynski and colleagues[2] also studied the intermetacarpal ligament anatomy. These investigators noted that the alignment of the interosseous ligaments between the fourth and fifth metacarpals differed from the ligament alignment between the second-third and third-fourth metacarpals, which allows a greater degree of motion in the fifth CMC joint (approximately 25° of flexion/extension) as compared with the fourth CMC joint (approximately 15°). It was also observed that when these metacarpals flex at the CMC joints, as in grasping, the dorsal interosseous ligament tightens and the anterior interosseous ligament relaxes. When the metacarpals extend at the CMC joints, the anterior ligament tightens and the posterior ligament relaxes, which retains a rigid interconnection between the bones.

An axial load to the fourth and fifth metacarpal heads secondary to a clenched-fist blow is often cited as the most common mechanism of injury of a fracture dislocation of the fifth carpometacarpal

[a] Los Angeles County Harbor-UCLA Medical Center, 1000 W. Carson Street, Torrance, CA 90502
[b] The Hand and Wrist Institute, 2808 Columbia Street, Torrance, CA 90503, USA
* The Hand and Wrist Institute, 2808 Columbia Street, Torrance, CA 90503, USA.
E-mail address: d-slutsky@msn.com

Hand Clin 27 (2011) 361–367
doi:10.1016/j.hcl.2011.05.010
0749-0712/11/$ – see front matter © 2011 Elsevier Inc. All rights reserved.

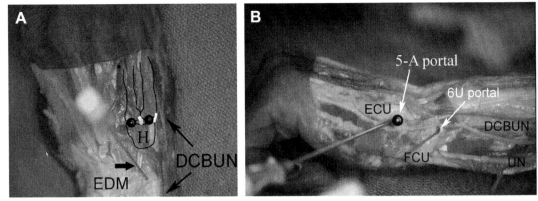

Fig. 1. (*A*) Cadaver dissection demonstrating the position of the two dorsal arthroscopy portals at the base of the fourth and fifth metacarpal bases (*radio buttons*) in relation to the metacarpohamate ligaments (in *white*). DCBUN (*arrows*), dorsal cutaneous branch of the ulnar nerve; EDM, extensor digiti minimi; H, hamate. (*B*) Lateral view demonstrating the position of the 5-A (accessory) portal relative to the 6U portal (*arrows*), which is located at the level of the fifth CMC joint, volar to the extensor carpi ulnaris (ECU). UN, ulnar nerve; FCU, flexor carpi ulnaris. (*Courtesy of* David J. Slutsky, MD, Los Angeles, CA.)

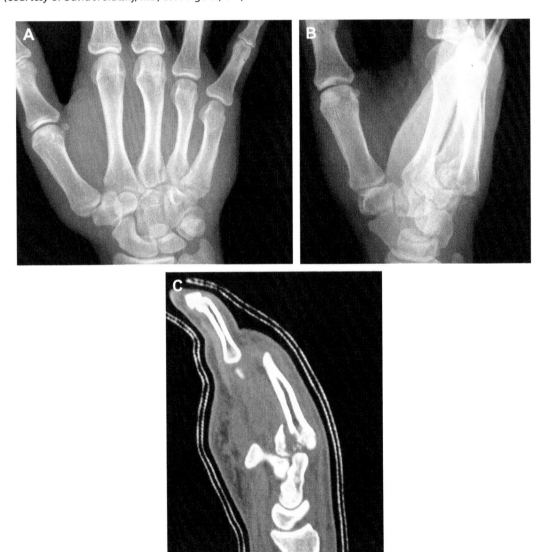

Fig. 2. (*A*) Anteroposterior view of a fracture dislocation of the fifth metacarpal CMC joint. (*B*) Lateral view shows the dorsal subluxation of the fifth metacarpal base as well as a comminuted dorsal hamate rim fracture. (*C*) Lateral computed tomography scan demonstrating the volar articular fragment. (*Courtesy of* David J. Slutsky, MD, Los Angeles, CA.)

joint. In one clinical study the investigators postulated that flexion during impact results in a dorsal dislocation of the small finger MC base, dorsal CMC ligament disruption, and often a hamate dorsal rim fracture.[3] Yoshida and colleagues[4] attempted to reproduce the mechanism of injury in a cadaver study by dropping an 8-kg weight from various heights onto the fourth and fifth metacarpal heads in a specially designed jig. The hand was placed in the clenched-fist position with the ring CMC joint in 20° of flexion, the small CMC joint in 30° of flexion, and the wrist in 20° of extension. A dorsal hamate fracture occurred in 45% of the specimens, whereas a fracture of the volar aspect of the ring and small finger MC base were present in 40% and 20% of the specimens, respectively. The small metacarpal volar base fracture fragment remained attached to the ring MC ulnar-side base–small MC radial-side base ligament.

IMAGING

Anteroposterior and lateral radiographs do not allow for an accurate assessment because the ring and small CMC joints are obscured by overlap of the hamate on the MC bases. Cain and colleagues[3] noted that a 45° pronation oblique view allowed for a good assessment of injuries to both the ring and small joints. Occasionally a 15° pronation oblique projection is required to assess damage to the dorsal portion of the small finger CMC joint.[4]

EQUIPMENT AND IMPLANTS

In general, a 2.7-mm 30° angled scope along with a camera attachment is used, although a 1.9-mm scope can be substituted. A 3-mm hook probe is needed for palpation of intracarpal structures.

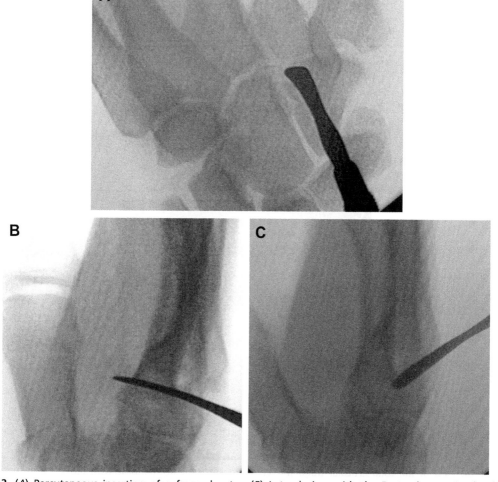

Fig. 3. (*A*) Percutaneous insertion of a freer elevator. (*B*) Lateral view with the Freer elevator in the fifth CMC joint. (*C*) Percutaneous reduction of the dorsal subluxation of the fifth metacarpal base. (*Courtesy of David J. Slutsky, MD, Los Angeles, CA.*)

At least 10 to 15 lb (4.5–6.8 kg) of traction is crucial to the success of the procedure, with either a traction tower or some other type of overhead traction. A motorized 2.9-mm full-radius resector is needed for debridement of hematoma, as well as small curettes and a dental hook for manipulation of the fracture fragments. The procedure is done with a fluoroscopic assist.

SURGICAL TECHNIQUE

The patient is positioned supine on the operating table with the arm extended on a hand table. The small and ring fingers are suspended by Chinese finger traps with 10 to 15 lb of countertraction.

The relevant landmarks are outlined including the proximal and dorsal edge of the fifth metacarpal base, the extensor carpi ulnaris (ECU) tendon, and if possible the extensor tendons to the small and ring fingers. The procedure is performed with a tourniquet elevated to 250 mm Hg. It is the author's preference to use a dry technique with intermittent saline irrigation through the scope, using a 10-mL syringe and suction using the full-radius resector, akin to the technique described by del Pinal and colleagues[5] for wrist arthroscopy. Two main portals are used (**Fig. 1**). There is an ulnar portal or fifth metacarpohamate portal (5-MH), which is located between the fifth MC ulnar-side base–hamate ligament and the extensor digiti

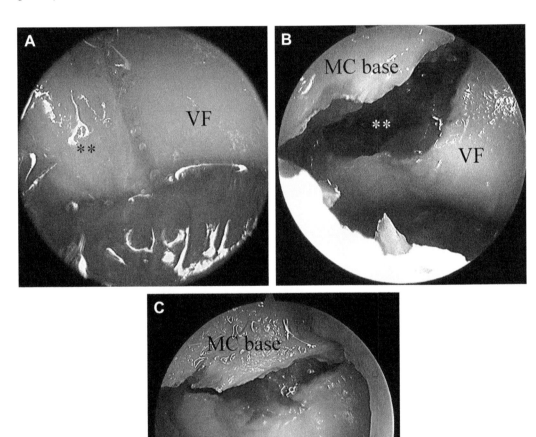

Fig. 4. (A) View of the volar articular fragment (VF) of the fifth metacarpal base with the scope in the 4-MH portal demonstrating the attached intermetacarpal ligament (asterisks). (B) The fracture gap (asterisks) is visualized by angling the scope dorsally and distally. MC base, dorsal metacarpal base. (C) Reduction of the fracture gap. (Courtesy of David J. Slutsky, MD, Los Angeles, CA.)

quinti tendon, at the level of CMC joint. The radial portal, or the fourth metacarpohamate portal (4-MH), is just radial to the fourth MC ulnar-side base–hamate ligament extensor tendon to the ring finger. Each joint is localized with a 22-gauge needle followed by injection of 2 mL of saline. This step may be facilitated by fluoroscopy. A small transverse skin incision is made followed by wound-spread technique with tenotomy scissors. The capsule is pierced and a cannula and blunt trocar are inserted, followed by the arthroscope. The portals are interchangeably used to systematically inspect the joint, which is facilitated by judicious use of a 2.9-mm resector. An accessory portal (5-A) can facilitate triangulation, located along the ulnar base of the fifth metacarpal just dorsal to the hypothenar muscles and approximately 1 cm distal to the 6-U wrist arthroscopy portal. There is no internervous plain, and injury to the dorsal cutaneous branch of the ulnar nerve is a risk with all of these portals; hence, careful wound-spread technique is mandatory. **Fig. 2** shows the characteristic radiographic appearance of a fracture subluxation of the fifth CMC joint. The dorsal subluxation of the fifth metacarpal base can be reduced by inserting a Freer elevator through the 5-MH portal at the base of the fifth metacarpal (**Fig. 3**). The 4-MH portal is established as described, followed by insertion of the blunt trocar and cannula and then the arthroscope. A 2.9-mm full-radius resector is inserted through the 5-MH portal and interchanged with a curette for debridement of the fracture debris. The 4-MH can be used as the viewing portal with the 5-MH as the working portal. A 0.045-inch (1.1 mm) K-wire can be inserted into the volar articular fragment and the metacarpal base, and used to manipulate the fragments. The volar articular fragment often remains attached to the fourth metacarpal base through an intact intermetacarpal ligament (**Fig. 4**). This attachment prevents displacement of the volar articular fragment, similar to the Bennett fracture fragment, which remains attached to the first intermetacarpal ligament. A useful maneuver is to pull the volar articular fragment dorsally with the dental pick while pushing volarly on the metacarpal base, to reduce the fracture gap. Prepositioned K-wires inserted in both of the fracture fragments are then advanced to capture the reduction. It is often necessary to cross-pin the fifth CMC joint to the hamate or capitate for 4 to 6 weeks to prevent recurrent dorsal subluxation (**Fig. 5**).

POSTOPERATIVE MANAGEMENT

The small and ring fingers are immobilized in a finger spica splint for 4 weeks, followed by protected finger motion. If the fixation is stable, passive and active MP joint flexion can be instituted early on. The K-wires are removed at 6 weeks. Strengthening ensues once motion has been restored. Clenched-fist striking, contact sports, and ball sports are allowed at 12 weeks

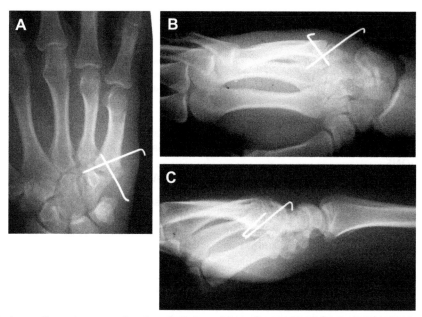

Fig. 5. (A) Postoperative anteroposterior view demonstrating and anatomic reduction of the fracture fragments. (B) Oblique view (15° pronation) highlighting the reduction of the dorsal subluxation of the fifth metacarpal base. (C) Lateral view showing a congruent joint reduction. (*Courtesy of* David J. Slutsky, MD, Los Angeles, CA.)

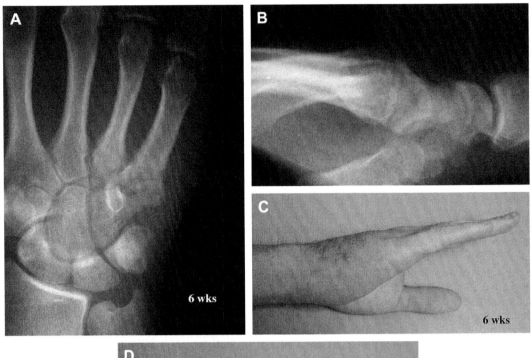

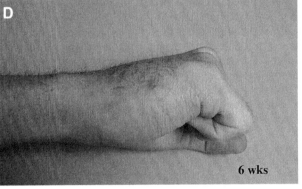

Fig. 6. (*A*) Anteroposterior view 6 weeks after K-wire removal, showing an anatomic union of the fracture fragments. (*B*) Lateral view demonstrating maintenance of the joint reduction. (*C, D*) Clinical photographs demonstrating normal finger range of motion at 6 weeks. (*Courtesy of* David J. Slutsky, MD, Los Angeles, CA.)

but may be permitted sooner if a playing cast or orthosis is used.

COMPLICATIONS

Potential complications of this procedure include injury to the dorsal cutaneous branch of the ulnar nerve, which cloaks the operative field. Direct or indirect extensor tendon injury or postoperative extensor tendon adhesions can be minimized by careful operative technique during the establishment of the portals and insertion of the K-wires, and by the institution of early finger motion. Iatrogenic articular damage can be minimized by using small joint instruments and joint distraction. Recurrent dorsal subluxation of the fifth metacarpal base can be minimized by temporary K-wire fixation of

the fifth CMC joint to allow ligamentous healing as well as internal fixation of any significant-sized dorsal hamate rim fractures.

SUMMARY

Early results with this procedure are encouraging (**Fig. 6**). The technique of small joint arthroscopy is especially useful because the fifth metacarpal volar articular fragment can usually only be visualized by retraction of the dorsal metacarpal base, which can be quite arduous. In addition, once the fracture fragments are reduced through an open incision the fracture lines can no longer be directly visualized without forceful manual distraction of the fifth metacarpal. The use of arthroscopy provides a magnified view of the fracture line as well as the ability to directly visualize the quality of the articular reduction. Akin to other joints, however, an anatomic reduction of the articular surface is desirable, but there are no data to establish that this results in improved clinical outcomes. Long-term follow-up is unavailable as yet, hence this procedure should be viewed as a useful adjunctive technique in the treatment of a fracture dislocation of the fifth CMC joint, but it is unlikely to supplant the more time-tested open procedures.

REFERENCES

1. Nakamura K, Patterson RM, Viegas SF. The ligament and skeletal anatomy of the second through fifth carpometacarpal joints and adjacent structures. J Hand Surg Am 2001;26:1016–29.
2. Dzwierzynski WW, Matloub HS, Yan JG, et al. Anatomy of the intermetacarpal ligaments of the carpometacarpal joints of the fingers. J Hand Surg Am 1997;22:931–4.
3. Cain JE Jr, Shepler TR, Wilson MR. Hamatometacarpal fracture-dislocation: classification and treatment. J Hand Surg Am 1987;12:762–7.
4. Yoshida R, Shah MA, Patterson RM, et al. Anatomy and pathomechanics of ring and small finger carpometacarpal joint injuries. J Hand Surg Am 2003;28: 1035–43.
5. del Pinal F, Garcia-Bernal FJ, Pisani D, et al. Dry arthroscopy of the wrist: surgical technique. J Hand Surg Am 2007;32:119–23.

Metacarpophalangeal Joint Arthroscopy: Indications Revisited

Alexander K.Y. Choi, MBChB, FRCS(Edinburgh), FRCSEd(Ortho), FHKCOS, FHKAM(Orthopaedic Surgery)[a,*],
Esther C.S. Chow, MBBS, MRCS(Edin), MMSc, FRCSEd(Ortho)[b,c],
P.C. Ho, MBBS, FRCS(Edinburgh), FHKCOS, FHKAM(Orthopaedic Surgery)[b,c], Y.Y. Chow, MBBS, FRCS(Edin), FRACS, FHKCOS, FHKAM(Orthopaedic Surgery)[a,c]

KEYWORDS

- Metacarpophalangeal • Arthroscopy • Thumb • Finger

Arthroscopic surgery has become the gold standard for the diagnosis and treatment of major joint disorders. With advancement in arthroscopic technique, arthroscopy has become feasible in most human joints, even those as small as the finger joints. The metacarpophalangeal joint (MCPJ) is an ideal joint for performing arthroscopic surgery. This joint can become spacious with simple traction. Moreover, the intra-articular anatomy is simple and its major structures can be easily visualized and identified. However, MCPJ arthroscopy has never been popularized. Arthroscopy of finger joints was first described in 1979.[1] Since then, there have been fewer than 10 reports on this subject published in the literature. This article describes our experience with MCPJ arthroscopy and seeks to establish its role in clinical practice.

ANATOMY OF THE MCPJ
The Finger MCPJ

The normal MCPJ is a diarthrodial, condylar-type joint that allows movement in multiple directions including flexion, extension, radial deviation, ulnar deviation, and circumduction. The metacarpal head is asymmetrical in both the coronal and sagittal planes. The radial condyle of the metacarpal head is larger than the ulnar condyle, which causes the metacarpal head to slope ulnarly in the coronal plane, especially in the second and third MCPJs. The volar surface of the metacarpal head is longer and broader than its dorsal surface, which accounts for the cam effect that tightens the collateral ligaments when the joint is flexed. The normal synovial membrane of the MCPJ is attached around the periphery of the articular cartilage with volar and dorsal synovial reflections. The synovial fold is largest dorsally on the neck of the metacarpal. The volar plate supports the MCPJ volarly and it consists of a membranous part and a cartilaginous part. The membranous portion of the volar plate attaches to the metacarpal neck and has more laxity than its distal insertion. The cartilaginous portion of the volar plate is distal and attaches firmly to the base of the proximal phalanx. The volar plates of adjacent digits are interconnected by the

This work was in part supported by a research grant of the Hong Kong College of Orthopaedic Surgeons (2003 to 2004). The authors have nothing to disclose.
[a] Department of Orthopaedics & Traumatology, Tuen Mun Hospital, 23 Tsing Tsun Koon Road, Tuen Mun, NT, Hong Kong SAR, China
[b] Department of Orthopaedics & Traumatology, Prince of Wales Hospital, 30-32 Ngan Shing Street, Shatin, NT, Hong Kong SAR, China
[c] Department of Orthopaedics & Traumatology, Faculty of Medicine, The Chinese University of Hong Kong, 30-32 Ngan Shing Street, Shatin, NT, Hong Kong SAR, China
* Corresponding author.
E-mail address: alexcatchoi@yahoo.com

Hand Clin 27 (2011) 369–382
doi:10.1016/j.hcl.2011.05.007

fibers of the deep transverse intermetacarpal ligament. The radial and ulnar collateral ligaments, which lie dorsal to the center of rotation of the MCPJ, reinforce the joint. These ligaments are lax when the joint is extended and become taut when the joint is flexed.

The Thumb MCPJ

The basic anatomy of MCPJ of the thumb is similar to that in the finger. However, compared with MCPJ of fingers, only a minor degree of movement in radioulnar plane and rotation is possible because of the greater stiffness of the collateral ligaments, which are important in providing stability to the thumb. There is also great variation in its range of movement between individuals and also between left and right.[2,3] This variation may be related to different shapes of the metacarpal head.[4] People with stiffer metacarpal joints in their thumbs are slightly more prone to injury.[2]

The presence of sesamoids also represents another difference from finger MCPJ. The sesamoids lie within the lateral and medial margin of the volar plate and at the origin of the fibroosseous sheath of the flexor pollicis longus tendon. The accessory collateral ligament inserts into the peripheral margin of the sesamoid on each side. The tendon of the adductor pollicis inserts onto the ulnar sesamoid, whereas the tendon of flexor pollicis brevis inserts onto the radial sesamoid.

Arthroscopic Anatomy

In the arthroscopic view, the appearance of thumb and finger MCPJ is similar. There are several consistent anatomic landmarks inside the MCPJ **(Fig. 1)**. These landmarks include (1) the radial

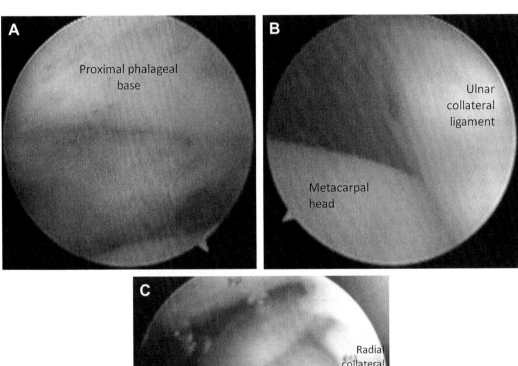
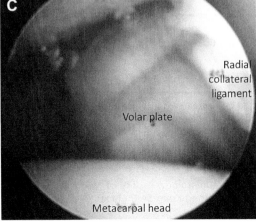

Fig. 1. (A) Intra-articular anatomy: proximal phalanx base. (B) Intra-articular anatomy: ulnar collateral ligament. (C) Intra-articular anatomy: radial collateral ligament.

and ulnar collateral ligaments that run obliquely from the metacarpal head to the proximal phalanx base; (2) 4 synovial recesses (radial, ulnar, volar, dorsal); (3) metacarpal head, which is wider at the volar end than the dorsal end; (4) proximal phalanx base; and (5) the volar plate. In the thumb, the sesamoid-metacarpal articulation is not usually visible. Although the MCPJ is readily distensible and allows free access for arthroscopy, there remains a blind spot in the joint that is inaccessible, which is the volar recess (**Fig. 2**) between the volar plate and the volar aspect of the metacarpal head. This volar recess may be partially accessed with the finger in flexion. In the thumb, the volar recess can be reached by probe or Freer when release of adhesion between the volar plate and the metacarpal head is required.

IMAGING

Plain radiographs provide a lot of information that is needed for diagnosis and formulating treatment plans for any lesions of the thumb MCPJ. In addition, stress views, flexion-extension views, fluoroscopy, and arthrogram may add additional information to the integrity of the collateral ligament or the volar plate.

Stress view of the thumb MCPJ is performed with thumb in extension in the anteroposterior view. The criteria to suggest complete collateral ligament tear varies from 30° to 45°.[5] The lack of end point or laxity significantly greater than the opposite side is another clue.

Static true lateral views of thumb in flexion and extension or fluoroscopy provide important information to assess the congruity of the MCPJ. A true lateral view of a normal MCPJ of the thumb is obtained when both sesamoids maximally overlap each other. In a normal thumb in neutral extension, the dorsal cortex of the proximal phalanx should be in line with the dorsal cortex of first metacarpal. On flexion, the proximal phalanx rotates concentrically over the center axis of the metacarpal head and the 2 sesamoids overlap throughout the range indicating no rotation from extension to flexion. We have performed a fluoroscopic study with 20 normal thumbs to assess such congruity on flexion and noticed that, at 30 to 40 degrees of flexion, the contour of volar cortex of the proximal phalanx forms a smooth, continuous line with that of the metacarpal in 18 out of 20 normal thumbs (**Fig. 3**A). This continuity is analogous with the Shenton line in the hip. In the remaining 2 patients, the lateral profile of the metacarpal head was flattened and beaked in shape.

In complete tear or high-grade laxity of one of the collateral ligaments, apparent volar subluxation or translation of proximal phalanx over the metacarpal head can be observed on static extension view (**Fig. 4**). This extension incongruity is caused by concomitant dorsal ligament tears with malrotation of the joint and the sesamoids not overlapping.[5,6]

However, in patients suffering from chronic pain after a sprain of the thumb MCPJ without significant collateral laxity, we have observed that there is loss of flexion congruity. The proximal phalanx apparently translates rather than rotates congruently over the metacarpal head while the sesamoids remain well overlapped. This condition results in the broken continuity of the volar cortices of the metacarpal and proximal phalanx on flexion. There is no malrotation observed in these cases. This phenomenon has not been reported before and is observed in about 80% of patients presented to us with chronic pain after sprain (see **Fig. 3**B). In more severe cases, this volar translation also persists on extension.

When performed in such a patient, a contrast arthrogram shows contracted volar recesses of the thumb MCPJ compared with the normal opposite side (**Fig. 5**). Intervening filling defects may also be observed, presumably representing fibrous adhesions. No contrast leakage was observed in any direction. This phenomenon can be reproduced in cadaveric specimens. When the volar plate is tethered to the metacarpal head by pins, volar translation of the proximal phalanx occurs on flexion (**Fig. 6**). We postulate that the obliteration of volar recess is the reason why the proximal phalangeal base cannot rotate congruently over the metacarpal head on flexion. This secondary incongruity may be the source of chronic pain and release of the volar recess may provide a cure.

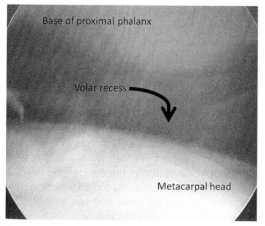

Base of proximal phalanx

Volar recess

Metacarpal head

Fig. 2. Volar recess and proximal part of volar plate: cannot be fully visualized arthroscopically.

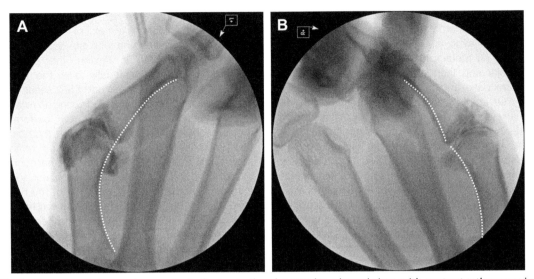

Fig. 3. Normal and abnormal congruity in flexion in thumb MCPJ (true lateral view, with contrast arthrogram injected in this case). (*A*) Normal flexion: volar cortices of metacarpal and proximal phalangeal shaft form a smooth arc (*dotted line*). (*B*) Abnormal flexion with broken arc (*dotted line*) of the metacarpal and proximal phalanx, suggesting incongruent flexion caused by volar translation. L+, left side; R+, right side.

Sophisticated imaging like ultrasonography, bone scintigraphy, computed tomography, and magnetic resonance imaging (MRI) is seldom of use in our practice. They are mainly indicated for preoperative diagnosis of Stener lesion, exclusion of occult fracture or osteochondral lesion, and assessment of neoplastic lesion.

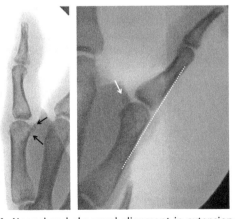

Fig. 4. Normal and abnormal alignment in extension of thumb MCPJ. In this patient, the left thumb with a complete ulnar collateral ligament tear shows volar translation on extension. The sesamoid do not overlap on an apparently true lateral view (*black arrows*). The normal right thumb shows no volar translation and the dorsal cortices of proximal phalanx and metacarpal are in line with each other (*white dotted line*). The sesamoids overlap well (*white arrow*).

GENERAL TECHNIQUE OF MCPJ ARTHROSCOPY

The procedure can be performed on an outpatient basis with portal-site local anesthesia or regional anesthesia. The patient is placed in a supine position with shoulder abducted and the arm supported on an arm board (**Fig. 7**). No tourniquet is required. The instruments used include 1.9-mm arthroscope (30° lens), 2.0-mm shaver, Mini-VAPR (Depuy Mitek, Raynham, MA, USA), mini-Vulcan (Smith & Nephew, Andover, MA, USA), and mini arthroscopic instruments (**Fig. 8**). A finger trap is applied to the affected finger. Plastic is preferred to metal for patient's maximal comfort. Traction is applied at 2.5 to 4.5 kg of tension with a traction tower. A 2-portal technique is used, a dorsal-radial portal and a dorsal-ulnar portal, one on either side of the central extensor tendon (**Figs. 9** and **10**). Once in traction, the vacuum sign becomes apparent and the joint space can easily be determined by thumb palpation. The intended port sites are marked with a marking pen. Local anesthesia with 1 to 1.5 mL of 2% lignocaine admixed with 1:200,000 adrenaline is injected to the port sites with a fine 26-G needle from the skin down to the level of the joint capsule. Intra-articular injection is optional and the needle can be used to confirm the joint space. Two milliliters of normal saline are injected via either port site for distention of the joint space. A longitudinal or oblique incision along the skin crease of less than 0.5 cm is made with a no.15 blade. The subcutaneous tissue is

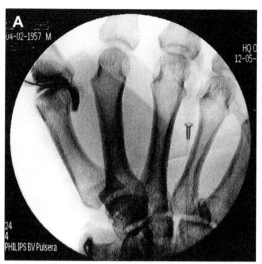
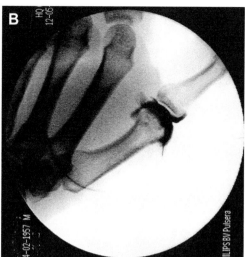

Fig. 5. Contrast arthrogram of thumb MCPJ. (*A*) A normal volar recess is spacious. (*B*) In patient with chronic pain after sprain, it may be contracted with little contrast retention. A similar illustration can also be found in **Fig. 2**.

dissected and extensor expansion is perforated by blunt dissection with a fine mosquito artery forceps. Joint space is confirmed once the gush of saline fluid egressed. Next, a cannula with a blunt or tapered end trocar is introduced into the dorsal-radial portal. Gentle force should be used to avoid scraping the articular cartilage of the metacarpal head, particularly in a tight joint. The trocar is then removed. Continuous saline infusion using 3 L of normal saline bag under gravity is connected to the cannula. Saline solution is allowed to fill the joint and the cannula before the arthroscope is inserted to avoid trapping an air bubble inside the joint. The dorsal-ulnar portal is used for instrumentation if it is a right hand. However, the 2 portals are interchangeable. If arthroscopy is done for a left hand, the 2 portals are reversed, that is, the dorsal-ulnar portal is used for the arthroscope and the dorsal-radial portal is used for the instruments. It is recommended to use the finger pivoting technique with the index or middle finger tip to fine control the lens motion because the joint is small and shallow. It is particularly important in dealing with dorsal sided disorders, such as chondral lesion or synovitis, to avoid the frequent dislodgement of the arthroscope.

The MCPJ is a simple joint to examine arthroscopically because there is only 1 joint space. With the 30° arthroscope inside the joint, the dome-shaped cartilaginous surface of the metacarpal

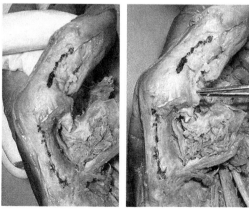

Fig. 6. Simulation of flexion incongruity in cadaver by tethering the volar plate to the metacarpal head by pins.

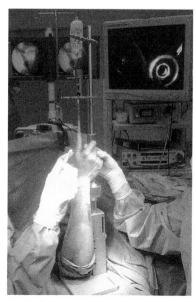

Fig. 7. Surgical setup.

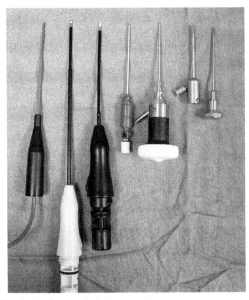

Fig. 8. Arthroscopic instruments.

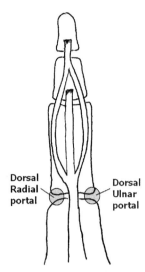

Fig. 10. Dorsal-radial and dorsal-ulnar portals as shown.

head should be apparent on the floor, whereas part of the concave articular surface of the base of the proximal phalanx can be seen in the upper part of the view. The volar plate can be seen between the 2 articular surfaces. However, the volar recess cannot be visualized normally because of its anterior and proximal location relative to the head. A probe can be inserted from the dorsoulnar portal to palpate

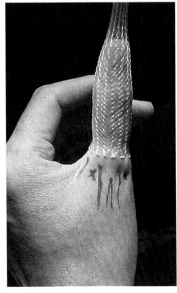

Fig. 9. Dorsal-radial and dorsal-ulnar portals.

the recess. By rotating the lens through 360°, a much wider area of the articular surfaces can be reached. The dorsal part of the metacarpal head and the accompanying dorsal synovial recess and capsular reflection can be seen with the lens facing downward. It is important to assess this part of the joint because many painful chondral lesions tend to be located in this area, together with the associated synovitis. The synovitis needs to be debrided with a 2-mm shaver to reveal the true extent of any chondral lesion. Alternatively a radiofrequency apparatus with the miniprobe is equally effective. However, a thermal phone at the dorsal side of the joint should be used with extreme caution because of the proximity to the extensor mechanism. Over the volar plate area, the long flexor tendon is also at risk of thermal damage. Toward the radial side, the arthroscope can follow the articular surface of the metacarpal head to sweep into the radial gutter to reach the radial synovial recess where the radial collateral ligament originates. The ligament can be assessed for any substance tear, avulsion, or laxity, and any loose body can be removed. It may be difficult to see the ulnar gutter and ulnar synovial recess from the radial side and the arthroscope needs to be inserted from the dorsoulnar portal to have a more thorough assessment.

After the procedure, the skin wounds are apposed with sterile strip and bulky dressings are applied for 2 days. The postoperative mobilization varies for different patients based on the underlying disorder. Patients with acute collateral ligament tears are immobilized after the operation, otherwise patients are encouraged to start free mobilization exercise as soon as pain allows.

INDICATIONS
Arthritis

Inflammatory arthritis

As suggested in previous reports, MCPJ arthroscopy is useful in revealing cartilage changes and synovial proliferation with minimal morbidity in rheumatoid hands.[7,8] Moreover, synovial biopsy and synovectomy can be performed without the need of an arthrotomy. In our series, arthroscopic synovectomy has been performed in 8 cases of inflammatory arthritis (1 rheumatoid arthritis, 5 psoriatic arthritis, 2 seronegative arthritis) with good symptomatic relief. This technique also allows tissue biopsy for more detailed histologic study in cases in which the diagnosis of inflammatory arthritis has not yet been established. In severe cases, the arthroscopic views are frequently obscured by the dense synovial overgrowth inside the joint. The detail architecture of the joint may not be apparent at the beginning. It is mandatory to start shaving synovium with a small shaver, even with limited vision, to reveal more articular structure. Usually the view is improved after some debridement of synovium. The status of the articular cartilage should be documented on both sides of the joint. The morphology of the synovial overgrowth may also help to differentiate the underlying disorder. A villonodular appearance signifies inflammatory arthritis. A chalky tophaceous material deposition can be seen in gouty arthritis. A fibrinoid appearance may suggest infective origin. A posttraumatic lesion is usually fibril-like. The application is particularly valuable in managing monoarthritis or oligoarthritis, both for diagnostic and therapeutic effect. In our series, a 49-year-old woman presented with right ring finger swelling and pain for 10 months. The blood tests for rheumatoid factors and antinuclear antibody were negative. We performed a MCPJ arthroscopy that revealed severe synovitis and synovial overgrowth within the joint with preserved articular cartilage. The differential diagnosis included chronic infection such as tuberculosis or fungal infection, rheumatoid arthritis, and other inflammatory arthritis. A synovial biopsy was taken for molecular study of tuberculosis DNA, which was negative. The culture results were also negative. The pathology report confirmed chronic inflammation and the patient was later diagnosed as having psoriasis. The skin lesion became apparent later and she was placed in the care of a rheumatologist.

Although arthroscopic synovectomy is effective in providing symptomatic relief, it may not be possible to alter the disease progress in cases of inflammatory arthritis. As a result, the symptoms may recur with increased synovial overgrowth and periarticular erosions. In our series, 3 cases required secondary procedures after an initial period of symptom relief. One case required a fusion 6 years after the initial arthroscopy, and 2 cases required an arthroplasty 1 year after the initial arthroscopic surgery.

Osteoarthritis

The role of MCPJ arthroscopy is less well established in patients with osteoarthritis and is mainly for diagnostic purposes. None of the other diagnostic or imaging modalities, even MRI, can provide detailed and accurate information regarding the integrity of the cartilage surfaces of the MCPJ.

There was only 1 case of osteoarthritis in our series and the arthroscopic findings showed severe osteochondral defects on both joint surfaces. Pain relief was unsatisfactory after the initial arthroscopy and this patient required a pyrocarbon arthroplasty 1 year after the initial arthroscopic surgery.

Acute Trauma

Acute collateral ligaments injury/gamekeeper's thumb

The use of MCPJ arthroscopy for the treatment of gamekeeper's thumb was first described by Ryu and Fagan[9] in 1995. However, this technique has not become widely used. Although the Stener lesion can be diagnosed with ultrasound or an MRI scan, these methods are less sensitive than direct visualization using the arthroscope. The role of MCPJ arthroscopy in cases of gamekeeper's thumb includes detection of a Stener lesion (**Fig. 11**A) and reduction of a Stener lesion if necessary. There are 2 cases of gamekeeper's thumb in our series and 1 of them had been confirmed to be a Stener lesion (see **Fig. 11**B, C). We were able to reduce the Stener lesion and reposition the ulnar collateral ligament back to its original position. The thumb was then immobilized with a cast for 4 weeks. The clinical outcome was good.

Reduction of metacarpal head fracture

Metacarpal head fractures are uncommon but are occasionally seen in young athletes. Frequently, the patient presents with mild swelling and a slight decrease in range of motion. The fracture may be missed if radiograph films are not well taken. Even with true anteroposterior and lateral radiograph films, the exact position of the fracture may not be well localized. MCPJ arthroscopy can be used for direct visualization to achieve an anatomic reduction of this difficult intra-articular fracture. The fracture can be fixed in a retrograde manner with an absorbable pin.

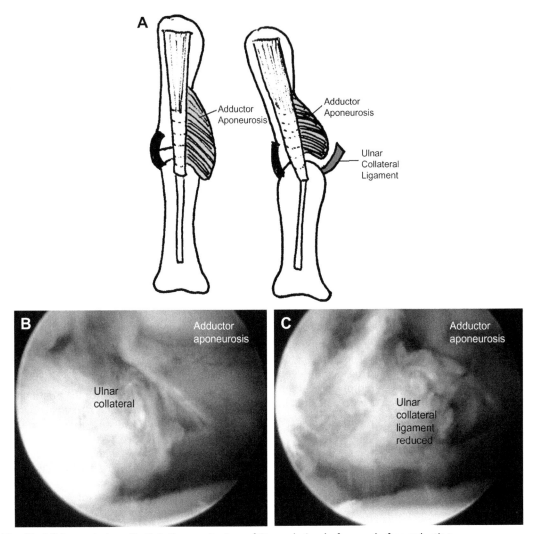

Fig. 11. (A) Stener lesion. (B, C) Arthroscopic view of Stener lesion before and after reduction.

Fig. 12 shows a case of right fourth metacarpal head intra-articular fracture after a sports injury. The patient was treated with MCPJ arthroscopic-assisted reduction under local anesthesia. With the aid of MCPJ arthroscopy, direct visualization of the fracture fragment was possible and the fracture fragment could be reduced using a probe. The fracture was then temporarily fixed with a 0.9-mm K-wire (**Figs. 13** and **14**) and then fixed with 2 absorbable pins in a retrograde manner (**Fig. 15**). After surgery, the patient was placed in a bulky dressing for 1 to 2 days and then allowed free mobilization as tolerated.

Complex MCPJ dislocation

MCPJ arthroscopy also plays an important role in patients with complex MCPJ dislocation. Reduction of the joint can be achieved with minimal surgical trauma, as in our series. There was 1

case of acute thumb MCPJ complex dislocation, which was caused by an entrapped sesamoid bone. The functional recovery was excellent.

Chronic Pain

Posttraumatic MCPJ pain of the thumb caused by fibrosis and volar plate adhesion

Sprained or incomplete collateral injuries are more common than complete collateral ligament tear. Such injuries are often missed and delayed in diagnosis.[10,11] In our experience, persistent pain and weakness of pinch after incomplete collateral injury is common. In our series, there were several patients suffering from persistent joint pain, especially during flexion after minor injuries. Conservative treatment with physiotherapy, splintage, and intra-articular steroid injection had failed. Although instability is not significant in this group of patients,

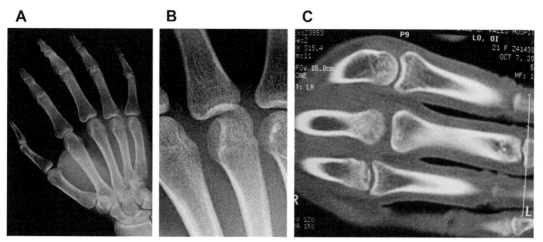

Fig. 12. (*A*) Fourth metacarpal head metacarpal fracture. (*B*) Fourth metacarpal head intra-articular fracture. (*C*) Computed tomography of the metacarpal head fracture.

the exact disorder leading to persistent symptoms is not known. In an early report by Vaupel and Andrews,[12] arthroscopy was used successfully to treat a patient with chronic painful synovitis and burring of small chondral defect.

Although dense synovitis, fibrosis, and osteochondral lesion are all common disorders encountered in such cases, volar plate adhesion leading to incongruent and painful flexion may be another important reason for chronic pain. In 15 cases, the patients were found to have volar plate adherent to the metacarpal head with obliteration of the volar recess. This condition was shown by an intraoperative arthrogram (see **Fig. 5**B) and resulted in incongruent flexion on fluoroscopy screening. The joint space was narrowed on introduction of the arthroscope. Synovectomy alone partially

opened the joint. It was fully released only after the volar plate adhesion broke down by insertion of a Freer dissector under direct vision (**Fig. 16**). The volar recess is thus reopened. Normal congruent flexion can be restored after surgery (**Fig. 17**). It was found to be a common phenomenon in patients with posttraumatic pain and stiffness in the thumb. Pain could be improved in all cases after such release.

Chrondral lesions

MCPJ arthroscopy is also useful for other intra-articular lesions, especially intra-articular cartilage defects. One study shows that MCPJ arthroscopy is more sensitive in the detection of intra-articular cartilage abnormalities compared with plain radiograph or MRI.[13] Such lesions may be sequelae to

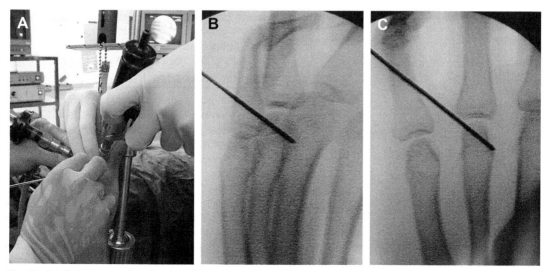

Fig. 13. (*A–C*) Arthroscopic reduction of metacarpal head fracture.

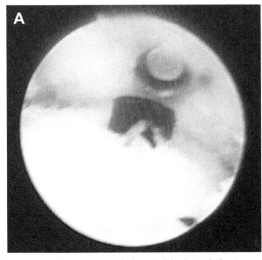
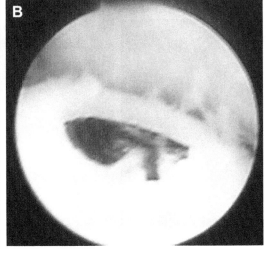

Fig. 14. (*A, B*) Insertion of absorbable (Vicryl©) pin.

the initial injury or secondary to incongruity. In the latter situation, the lesion is usually located over the dorsal aspect of the base of the proximal phalanx when it translates and hits over the metacarpal head on flexion. Pain improvement can be further achieved with debridement of the cartilage defects; however, pain control was not guaranteed. The prognosis depends on the severity of cartilage damage. One of the patients had a severe osteochondral defect over both the proximal phalanx base and the metacarpal head and required a secondary fusion.

There were 2 cases in our series with persistent pain and a mechanical block in the ring finger MCPJ caused by a previous missed metacarpal head fracture (see **Fig. 11**). A painful click was

felt inside the affected joint with movement. Intraoperative findings were similar in both cases and showed an unstable cartilage flap over the metacarpal head (see **Fig. 10**), whereas the collateral ligaments and synovium remained preserved. We were able to remove the unstable cartilage flap and smooth the joint surface. The mechanical block was relieved immediately and a good functional outcome was achieved.

Removal of loose bodies

Loose bodies are commonly seen in patients with inflammatory arthritis or in cases with posttraumatic cartilage damage. The symptoms can be disturbing, with pain and locking. MCPJ arthroscopy can be used to remove the loose bodies without significant surgical damage. Loose bodies are frequently lodged in synovial recesses, including radial, ulnar, and dorsal gutters. The volar plate recess is also commonly involved. Examination of the MCPJ is not complete without visualizing or probing into the recesses.

Chronic Instability

Patients with repeated thumb injury may suffer from thumb MCPJ instability with pain. Clinically the patient presents with pain at the extremes of motion. Capsular laxity and joint instability can be shown clinically with increased dorsal and volar translation associated with pain on examination. The use of a radiofrequency probe to induce thermal shrinkage of the joint capsule, especially the volar plate structure, can relieve the symptoms in such patients.

Thermal shrinkage had been commonly used in patients with shoulder instability. The thermal shrinkage technique involves the application of

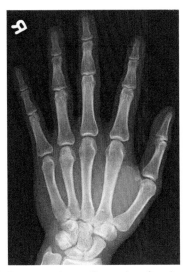

Fig. 15. Postoperative radiographs after healing of metacarpal fracture.

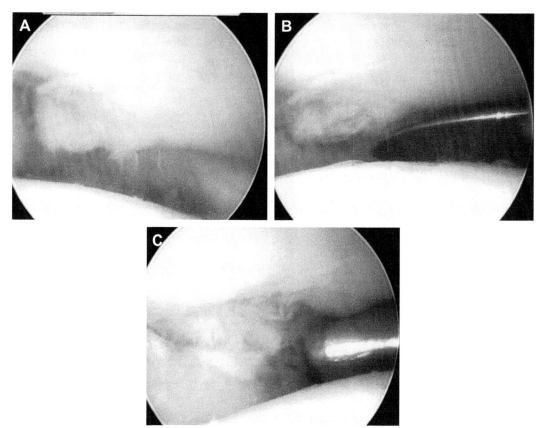

Fig. 16. Arthroscopic release of volar plate and volar recess. (*A*) Very narrowed joint space in a patient suffering from chronic pain and stiffness of thumb MCPJ after sprain. Synovitis has been partly debrided. (*B*) Insertion of a Freer dissector to release the adhesion between volar plate and metacarpal head by gently sliding in around the metacarpal head. (*C*) Joint space opened up after volar plate released and volar recess recreated.

heat using a specialized radiofrequency probe to shrink and tighten tissues. Tendons and ligaments are primarily composed of collagen. When collagen is heated to the appropriate temperature, it contracts and shrinks. The body perceives this as an injury and the tissues rebuild around shorter collagen fibers, resulting in a tighter, and theoretically more stable, joint. We borrowed this concept for the treatment of thumb MCPJ instability.

Several precautions are needed when using a radiofrequency probe: (1) intermittent transmission of radiofrequency signal should be used, instead of a continuous long duration of transmission; (2) continuous flow of irrigation fluid should be used. The reason for these precautions is to avoid overheating the surrounding structures, especially the flexor tendon and the neurovascular bundles, which are in close proximity to the volar capsule.

After surgery, the patient should be immobilized with a thumb spica slab for 3 to 4 weeks. Afterward, the patient is allowed to have free mobilization during the day time and must wear a thumb spica splint at night time.

Finger Stiffness

Stiffness without pain in the thumb MCPJ is well tolerated. However, MCPJ stiffness in fingers may be disabling. There are many causes of stiffness, both intra-articular and extra-articular. We selectively performed an arthroscopic release of a stiff MCPJ in 2 cases (1 middle finger and 1 little finger) caused by prolonged immobilization in an extended position with a subsequent loss of flexion. There was no preexisting injury in these 2 joints. Intraarticular fibrosis was removed arthroscopically and a limited extensor tenolysis was performed through the dorsal portals. The improvement in range of movement was satisfactory.

LIMITATIONS AND COMPLICATIONS

There is a limit to how fully the volar recess can be visualized. If the disorder of the MCPJ arises from extra-articular structures, such as an extensor synovitis, then MCPJ arthroscopy cannot be used to tackle the problem. Therefore, it is

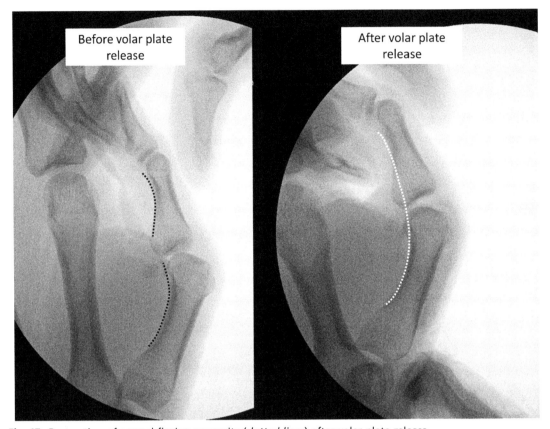

Fig. 17. Restoration of normal flexion congruity (*dotted lines*) after volar plate release.

essential to examine the patient carefully before the operation to differentiate intra-articular from extra-articular problems. Clinically, extensor synovitis tends to move with finger motion, whereas articular synovitis does not. These conditions can also be differentiated with ultrasonography or MRI before the operation. In cases of coexisting articular and extensor synovitis, an open extensor tenosynovectomy and an open arthroscopic synovectomy of the joint can be considered after the extensor mechanism is displayed and tenosynovitis surgically debrided.

Previous reports stated that maintaining distention of the joint is a major problem.[7,8,12] With adequate finger traction, the volume of the joint space is usually not a problem except in a very fibrotic and stiff joint. The use of continuous saline infusion helps to distend the dorsal synovial recess and aids the visual field in performing dorsal synovectomy.

POSSIBLE COMPLICATIONS
Wound Complication

Complications related to the wound are uncommon.

Complications Related to use of Radiofrequency Probes

Radiofrequency probes are commonly used for therapeutic purposes in MCPJ arthroscopy. However, there are known detrimental effects caused by heat production. Because the flexor tendons and the neurovascular bundles are in close proximity to the volar joint capsule, and because the joint capsule is thin, these structures are especially at risk of thermal damage. To minimize the thermal damage by using radiofrequency probes, special care must be taken and it must be used with adequate fluid lavage, for short durations, and use the minimal wattage as necessary.

We had 1 case of flexor pollicis longus rupture 3 weeks after thermal shrinkage of the volar plate. At the surgical exploration, the ruptured tendon ends were abnormal with a semitransparent appearance compatible with a thermal coagulation injury (**Fig. 18**). Histologic examination confirmed hyalinization of the collagen fibers, consistent with thermal damage. The volar plate instability was markedly improved after the shrinkage procedure. The ruptured tendon was treated with direct repair after excision of the abnormal segment. The

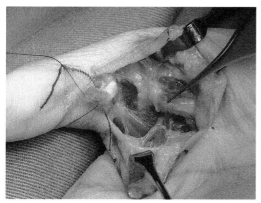

Fig. 18. Flexor pollicis longus rupture, presumably caused by thermal injury by radiofrequency probe.

outcome at 1 year showed normal range of motion of the thumb and complete resolution of pain and joint instability.

Tendon Injuries

The extensor tendons are at risk of damage because of their close proximity to the portal entry sites. To avoid damage to the extensor tendon, special care should be taken when entering the port sites and blunt dissection should be used to avoid damage. Because it is located adjacent to the volar recess, the flexor tendon is prone to damage by indirect thermal injury when using the radiofrequency probes.

Neurovascular Bundle Injury

Similar to the flexor tendon, the digital neurovascular bundles are in close proximity to the volar recesses. Therefore, they are prone to indirect thermal injury by the radiofrequency probes. The use of portal-site local anesthesia without tourniquet helps to preserved intact sensation of the finger during the surgery and hence provides useful patient feedback on any impaling injury to the neurovascular bundle.

Articular Cartilage Damage

The small volume of the joint poses risk to cartilage damage by the intra-articular manipulation. All maneuvers inside the joint must be gentle, without violence. No sharp instrument should be used.

CLINICAL RESULTS

We reviewed all patients who underwent MCPJ arthroscopy between December 1999 and December 2005 in 2 hospitals in Hong Kong (Prince of Wales Hospital and Tuen Mun Hospital). We had performed 34 MCPJ arthroscopies in 31 patients.

Twenty-two of 34 cases were for the thumb, 3 for the index finger, 5 for the middle finger, 3 for the ring finger, and 1 for the little finger. There were 20 male and 11 female patients with an average age of 40.7 years. Thirteen of 34 cases were performed under either local or regional anesthesia. The average operative time was 48.9 minutes. None of the cases had been converted to open surgery.

The indications for surgery included (1) posttraumatic pain (thumb = 15, finger = 4); (2) inflammatory arthritis (n = 8); (3) osteoarthritis (n = 1); (4) acute injury (n = 4); and posttraumatic stiffness (n = 2). The average duration of symptoms (excluding those with acute injury) was 17.2 months. Conservative treatment with physiotherapy, splintage, or intra-articular steroid injections had failed in all patients preoperatively. All patients were called back for a final follow-up. Whenever the patient was unable to come back for the final follow-up, the information was gathered via telephone interview and from case notes. Thirty of 31 patients were available for the final follow-up and the average follow-up period was 30 months (3–80 months). During the final follow-up, the patients were evaluated with objective measures, including range of motion, grip power, and pinch power. Clinical outcomes were also evaluated by pain score (visual analog scale), days before return to activities of daily living, and patient satisfaction. Case notes and operative records were reviewed and the intraoperative findings and the therapeutic procedures performed were studied. A statistical analysis using a paired t-test was performed with an online calculator (http://www.graphpad.com).

The overall patient satisfaction was excellent. The preoperative and postoperative pain scores (scale 0–10) were reported retrospectively during the final follow-up or from telephone interview. The differences in preoperative and postoperative pain scores were analyzed statistically with a paired t-test. The pain score improved from 6.8 before surgery to 2.44 after surgery ($P<.0001$), with a statistically significant difference. The range of motion of the affected MCPJ was compared with the contralateral side and analyzed by a paired t-test. The range of motion of the affected MCPJ averaged 62.3° (patients receiving either fusion or arthroplasty were excluded in this measurement). There was no significant difference between the affected side and the contralateral side (average = 67.5) with $P = .3535$. Similarly, a paired t-test was used to compare the grip power and pinch power of the affected side and contralateral normal side. The grip power of the affected side (mean = 27.7 kg) had no significant difference compared with the normal side (mean = 33.4 kg) with P = .0734. The pinch power of the affected side (mean = 5.6 kg) was comparable with the normal side (mean = 7.0 kg) with P = .0490. The time before return to activities of daily living ranged from 0 to 2 days.

In 5 cases, the symptomatic relief was temporary, the pain recurred after the initial procedure, and these cases required a secondary surgical procedure. These included (1) 1 case of left thumb post-traumatic osteochondral defects requiring a fusion 1 year after initial surgery; (2) 2 cases of psoriasis (index finger and middle finger) requiring arthroplasty 1 year after initial surgery; (3) 1 case of psoriasis of the thumb required fusion 6 years after surgery and (4) 1 case of osteoarthritis that required a pyrocarbon arthroplasty 6 months after surgery.

SUMMARY

MCPJ arthroscopy is a simple, safe, and effective procedure. It allows clear visualization of the intra-articular disorder with minimal soft tissue trauma. It provides satisfactory pain relief and good long-term functional outcome. The established roles of MCPJ arthroscopy include (1) synovectomy in inflammatory arthritis; (2) synovial biopsy in cases with uncertain diagnosis; (3) smoothening and debridement of cartilage flaps/fibrillations; (4) confirmation and reduction of a Stener lesion; (5) removal of loose bodies; (6) reduction of an entrapped sesamoid bone in an acute dislocation; and (7) release of an adherent volar plate in patients with persistent posttraumatic pain and stiffness. Other possible therapeutic procedures, including thermal shrinkage of joint capsules, are still being investigated. However, this is only a preliminary report and the indications of this technique should be revisited in the future.

REFERENCES

1. Chen YC. Arthroscopy of the wrist and finger joints. Orthop Clin North Am 1979;10:723–33.
2. Shaw SJ, Morris MA. The range of motion of the metacarpo-phalangeal joint of the thumb and its relationship to injury. J Hand Surg Br 1992;17:164–7.
3. Jenkins M, Bamberger HB, Black L, et al. Thumb joint flexion. What is normal? J Hand Surg Br 1998; 23:796–7.
4. Coonrad RN, Goldner JL. A study of the pathological findings and treatment in the soft-tissue injury of the thumb metacarpophalangeal joint. J Bone Joint Surg Am 1968;50:439–54.
5. Glickel SZ, Barton NJ, Eaton RJ. Dislocations and ligament injuries in the digit. In: Green DP, Hotchkiss RN, Pederson WC, editors. Green's operative hand surgery, vol. 2. 4th edition. Philadelphia: Churchill Livingstone; 1999. p. 772–808.
6. Smith RJ. Post-traumatic instability of the metacarpophalangeal joint of the thumb. J Bone Joint Surg Am 1977;59:14–21.
7. Sekiya I, Kobayashi M, Taneda Y. Arthroscopy of the proximal interphalangeal and metacarpophalangeal joints in rheumatoid hands. Arthroscopy 2002; 18(No.3):292–7.
8. Wei N, Delauter SK, Erlichman MS, et al. Arthroscopic synovectomy of the metacarpophalangeal joint in refractory rheumatoid arthritis: a technique. Arthroscopy 1999;15(No.3):265–8.
9. Ryu J, Fagan R. Arthroscopic treatment of acute complete thumb metacarpophalangeal ulnar collateral ligament tears. J Hand Surg Am 1995;20(No.6): 1037–42.
10. Carr D, Johnson RJ, Pope MH. Upper extremity injuries in skiing. Am J Sports Med 1981;9:378–83.
11. Miller RJ. Dislocations and fracture dislocations of the metacarpophalangeal joint of the thumb. Hand Clin 1988;4:45–65.
12. Vaupel GL, Andrews JR. Diagnostic and operative arthroscopy of the thumb metacarpophalangeal joint. A case report. Am J Sports Med 1985;13(No. 2):139–41.
13. Ostendorf B, Peters R, Dann P, et al. Magnetic resonance imaging and miniarthroscopy of metacarpophalangeal joints. Arthritis Rheum 2001;44(No.11): 2492–502.

New Frontiers in Hand Arthroscopy

Tyson K. Cobb, MD[a],*, Stacey H. Berner, MD[b],
Alejandro Badia, MD[c]

KEYWORDS

- Small joint arthroscopy • Trapeziometacarpal arthroscopy
- Thumb carpometacarpal arthroscopy
- Metacarpophalangeal arthroscopy
- Proximal interphalangeal joint arthroscopy
- Pisotriquetral joint arthroscopy
- Distal interphalangeal joint arthroscopic arthrodesis
- Metacarpophalangeal joint

This article covers new and emerging techniques in small joint arthroscopy in the hand. Recent improvement in the quality of small joint scopes and advancement in techniques have allowed for many new small joint arthroscopic procedures in the hand. The arthroscopic classification for thumb carpometacarpal (CMC) arthritis as well as treatment of each stage are covered. Findings for arthroscopic treatment of pantrapezial arthrosis are reviewed. Metacarpophalangeal (MCP) arthroscopy for the treatment of synovitis, arthritis, fractures, and gamekeeper injuries is discussed, as is arthroscopy of the proximal interphalangeal (PIP), pisotriquetral (PT), fourth and fifth CMC, and distal interphalangeal (DIP) joints.

ARTHROSCOPIC STAGING OF THUMB CMC JOINT

Arthroscopy allows for a true assessment of the joint status. Although thumb CMC arthritis has traditionally been staged by simple radiographic means,[1] this does not represent an accurate assessment of articular status. This observation is particularly true in the early stages of osteoarthritis, when symptoms are frequently worse than the radiographs suggest; an arthroscopic joint evaluation depicts the process.[2]

In arthroscopic stage I there is a diffuse synovitis but with minimal, if any, articular cartilage wear. Ligamentous laxity, particularly the volar ligaments, is a frequent finding. If the patient presents early enough, an arthroscopic synovectomy can be performed, using a full-radius resector and a radiofrequency probe, followed by shrinkage capsulorraphy if capsular redundancy is present. The joint is then protected in a thumb spica cast for several weeks depending on the extent of capsular laxity. A greater degree of joint instability requires a more aggressive capsulorraphy and longer immobilization to achieve joint stability and slow the progression of articular cartilage degeneration.

In arthroscopic stage II there is focal wear of the articular surface on the central to dorsal aspect of the trapezium and the deep palmar aspect of the metacarpal base. This situation does suggest that a progressive arthritic process is under way and requires a joint modifying procedure to alter the biomechanics of the joint. After an arthroscopic synovectomy, debridement, and frequent loose body removal, the joint is evaluated for any instability or laxity. A shrinkage thermal capsulorraphy

The authors have nothing to disclose.
[a] Orthopaedic Specialists, Davenport, IA, USA
[b] Advanced Centers for Orthopaedic Surgery and Sports Medicine, 10 Crossroads Drive Suite 210, Owings Mills, MD 21117, USA
[c] Badia Hand to Shoulder Center, Miami, FL, USA
* Corresponding author.
E-mail address: tysoncobbmd@gmail.com

is performed in many cases. The arthroscope is then removed and one of the portals is extended distally to approach the metacarpal base. A dorsoradial closing wedge osteotomy, akin to Wilson's original technique,[3] is then performed to place the thumb in an extended and abducted position.[4] This procedure is to minimize the tendency for metacarpal subluxation and to change the contact points of the worn articular cartilage, effectively centralizing the metacarpal. The osteotomy is usually stabilized by a single oblique K-wire that is also placed across the first CMC joint. Pinning allows for healing of the osteotomy in the correct position but also corrects the metacarpal subluxation that is often seen in this critical stage. Correction of the subluxation may arrest the arthritic process but there are no data to support this. A thumb spica cast protects the metacarpal during healing and the wire is removed 5 to 6 weeks after the operation. An arthroscopic staging is used to determine the ideal indications for this osteotomy, because it is difficult to determine which joints have early focal trapezial wear by any imaging modality. Metacarpal osteotomy has had good results in past studies, including a more recent paper by Tomaino.[5] Late follow-up of these patients has confirmed that the metacarpal remains centralized. The role of capsular shrinkage versus the alteration of force vectors by the use of osteotomy likely both play a role in changing the joint biomechanics.

In arthroscopic stage III there is diffuse trapezial articular cartilage loss. The metacarpal base may also show significant cartilage loss to varying degrees. The arthroscopic findings indicate that this is not a joint that is salvageable and a simple debridement or osteotomy does not provide an acceptable long-term result. An arthroscopic partial trapeziectomy is then performed by burring away the remaining articular cartilage and removing the subchondral bone down to a bleeding surface. This procedure functions not only to increase the joint space but to allow for cancellous bone bleeding, which forms a thrombus, becoming a fibrous tissue interposition. One might augment this procedure by inserting an interposition material, although superior results have not been proven with interposition.

Stage III can also be treated by a traditional open excisional arthroplasty, arthrodesis. or total joint replacement depending on surgeon preference. However, it has been our experience that the minimally invasive nature of arthroscopic resection arthroplasty has largely obviated open surgery, which is inherently more painful, more complication ridden, and limits future options.

Although arthroscopic management of Badia stage 1, 2, and 3 is an acceptable standard for many surgeons, patients with pantrapezial arthrosis have traditionally been treated with open procedures. Recently we have completed a study of 35 cases of arthroscopic resection arthroplasty performed at the scaphotrapeziotrapezoidal (STT) joint and the CMC for pantrapezial arthrosis with good results.[6]

Indications

Surgical indications include pain localized at both the CMC and STT joints, radiographic changes consistent with arthrosis, and full-thickness widespread cartilage loss of both joints found at the time of arthroscopy.

Contraindications

Contraindications include active infection and instability in patients who desire correction. In the authors' experience most patients are satisfied with pain relief despite persistent instability at the CMC and MCP joints.

Surgical Technique

The arm is suspended using 2.3 to 4.5 kg (5–10 pounds) of finger-trap traction on only the thumb. When indicated, diagnostic arthroscopy is performed with a 1.9-mm arthroscope. An arthroscopic resection arthroplasty is performed using a 2.3-mm or 2.7-mm arthroscope. Volar (1R) and dorsal (1U) portals are used for CMC arthroscopy. STT arthroscopy is performed through volar (1R) and dorsal (1U) portals, which are placed approximately 1 cm proximal to the corresponding CMC portals. An additional dorsal portal is used when necessary by placing a blunt probe through the volar portal across the STT or CMC joint and out the dorsum of the hand (**Fig. 1**).

Two to 3 mm of bone is removed from each side of both the CMC and STT joints with a 3.0-mm or 4.0-mm barrel bur (**Fig. 2**). Graft Jacket (Wright Medical Technology Inc, Arlington, TN, USA) was used as interposition material in 23 of the cases. The patients are typically immobilized for 1 to 3 weeks. The current protocol includes a postoperative splint for 1 week followed by a removable hand-based Orthoplast splint.

Preoperative data collected included a 2-point self-reported pain scale, disabilities of arm, shoulder and hand (DASH) outcome measure, range of motion, grip strength, and pinch strength.

Pain score (0–10) improved from 7 (range 5–10) preoperatively to 1 (range 0–6) at 1 year postoperatively (P<.0005) (**Fig. 3**). DASH score improved from 46 preoperatively to 19 at 1 year (**Fig. 4**).

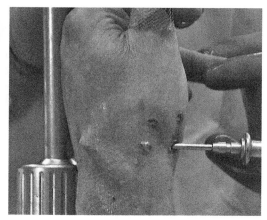

Fig. 1. Pantrapezial arthrosis: portal access across STT and CMC.

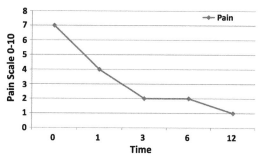

Fig. 3. Pantrapezial arthrosis: pain score improvement from preoperatively to 1 year postoperatively.

Thumb range of motion did not change significantly. All but one patient reached the base of the fifth digit at 1-year follow-up. The mean improvement in key pinch was 1.3 kg (2.9 pounds) (95% confidence internal [CI] 0.84–5.00) (P = .0008). The mean improvement in grip strength was 4.3 kg (9.52 pounds) (95% CI 1.467–17.56) (P = .023).

Complications

Two patients developed postoperative infections. One was superficial and resolved with outpatient antibiotics, and 1 deep infection required arthroscopic irrigation and debridement. Three patients developed a flexor carpi radialis tendonitis, 2 of which resolved with conservative treatment and

1 of which required surgical release. Two patients with persistent pain underwent open revision surgery. Five patients reported paresthesias in the distribution of the superficial branch of the radial nerve, all of which resolved by the third postoperative month.

MCP ARTHROSCOPY

The MCP joint is ideally suited for arthroscopic evaluation and treatment.[7–10] The neurovascular structures are not close to the arthroscopic portals. The bony and tendinous landmarks are generally easy to identify. The MCP joint represents a single compartment. Therefore, visualization and navigation of the joint are easily accomplished with a short learning curve. The indications, equipment, and technique associated with MCP arthroscopy are discussed in the next sections, supported with clinical case examples.

MCP arthroscopy is a useful diagnostic and therapeutic entity. There are several reports in the rheumatology literature of diagnostic staging of inflammatory arthropathy.[11–16] Synovectomy may be a useful adjunct in this patient population as well, with short-term improvement in symptoms. However, long-term benefits have not yet been established.[14] In addition, debridement, removal of loose bodies, and chondroplasty can be useful

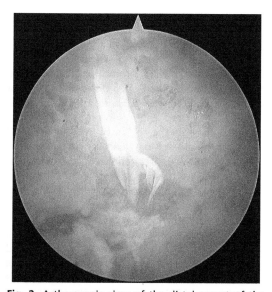

Fig. 2. Arthroscopic view of the distal aspect of the STT joint following arthroscopic resection.

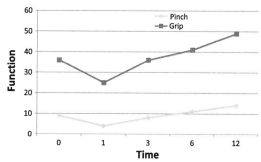

Fig. 4. Pantrapezial arthrosis: pinch and grip from pre-operatively to 1 year postoperatively.

in the posttraumatic setting.[10] Minimally invasive lavage and debridement can be performed in selected cases of intra-articular sepsis.

Arthroscopy can be useful for assessment and treatment of fractures, dislocations, and ligament injuries. Intra-articular fractures can be treated by arthroscopic and arthroscopically assisted means. Adequacy of reduction of the articular surface can be readily verified arthroscopically. Successful reduction of Stener lesions and arthroscopically assisted repair of collateral ligament injuries of the ulnar collateral ligament (UCL) of the thumb MCP joint have been reported within the literature.[17–22]

Expanded applications include arthrofibrectomy and arthroscopically assisted arthrodesis of thumb MCP joints. Current analysis of the feasibility of arthroscopically assisted arthroplasty may hold promise for the future.[7]

Equipment:

- Small joint arthroscope
- Traction apparatus
- Fluid management system
- Motorized shaver
- Small joint punch, grasper, biopsy forceps.

Optional:

- Currettes/osteotomes
- Fluoroscopy unit
- Wire driver
- Suture anchors
- Radiofrequency probe
- Headless screws.

Review of the literature reveals reports using various sizes and types of arthroscopes. The 1.0-mm needle arthroscope has been used for biopsy and staging procedures.[11,13] More commonly, the 1.7-mm, 1.9-mm, 2.0-mm, and 2.3-mm devices are used.[7,12,14,18] The authors' preference is a 1.9-mm, 30° arthroscope.

Various commercial traction tower devices are available. An overhead T-bar device (**Fig. 5**), is described in the technique section.

Normal saline or lactated Ringer solution can be used, at the surgeon's preference. An arthroscopic fluid pump can facilitate fluid management, provided that a low-pressure setting is used.

Technique

The patient is placed in the supine position and general or regional anesthesia is established. A pneumatic tourniquet is placed around the brachium of the operative extremity and an arm holder is applied. The arm holder attaches to the operating room bed and provides countertraction. An overhead T-bar is applied to the bed, directly

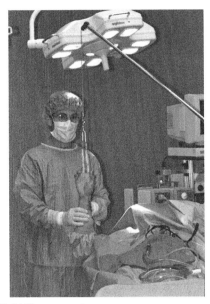

Fig. 5. MCP: scope set-up.

opposite the operative extremity. The hand and arm are prepared and draped in routine sterile fashion. A sterile finger trap is applied to the operative digit or thumb, and then attached to a hook on the T-bar. Sterile finger-trap application can be aided by the application of tincture of benzoin or Mastisol to the involved digit. Alternatively a K-wire may be inserted through the digit and finger trap to prevent slippage of the trap.[18] Weights are suspended from the opposite end of the pulley system in the T-bar. Traction of 4.5 kg (10 pounds) is applied through an overhead adjustable T-bar (see **Fig. 5**).

Radial and ulnar MCP portals are localized with the aid of 2 18-gauge needles (**Figs. 6** and **7**).

Fluoroscopic guidance may be used to assist in adequate identification of the joint space. The portals are established after distending the joint with 0.5% Marcaine or 0.9% normal saline solution. The radial and ulnar portals are each located off the midline, in the region of the sagittal hood fibers, in the interval between the collateral ligaments and the extensor tendon. In the digits the tubercles at the base of the proximal phalanges can be palpated and these represent the insertion points of the collateral ligaments. The extensor tendon is not violated. The skin is lanced and blunt dissection is performed until the joint capsule is encountered. A blunt arthroscopic trochar and cannula are inserted into the joint. The trochar is removed and the 1.9-mm, 30° arthroscope is placed in the MCP joint. Fluid inflow is through the arthroscope. An intravenous pressure bag is

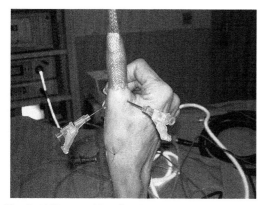

Fig. 6. MCP: portal localization.

applied to a 1-L bag of sterile 0.9% normal saline solution at 100 mm Hg. The pressure bag serves as a pump. Viewing and instrumentation portals are alternated. Small joint biopsy punches and graspers may be used. Debridement and synovectomy are performed with a 2.0-mm full-radius resector blade. Osteocartilagenous loose bodies are removed when encountered. A radiofrequency probe may be helpful to perform synovectomy and debridement, but care should be taken to provide adequate flow so as to avoid generating high temperatures in this low-volume joint. A monopolar probe may be preferable in this regard. Microcurrettes, elevators, and osteotomes may be useful for clearing debris, and performing manipulation of fragments during treatment of fractures. K-wires can be used as joysticks to assist in fracture reduction and may be used for provisional or definitive fracture fixation. Headless screws can be useful for treating large articular fracture fragments. These screws can be inserted percutaneously with arthroscopic and fluoroscopic guidance. Minisuture or microsuture anchors may be required for ligament repair.

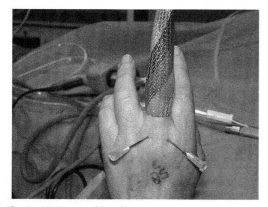

Fig. 7. MCP: portal localization.

Procedures and Illustrative Cases

Inflammatory arthropathy

Arthroscopy can be useful for staging and treatment of inflammatory arthropathy.[11–16,19,20] Synovectomy can be performed with a motorized shaver or a radiofrequency device. Maintenance of constant, but low-level inflow pressure provides adequate distention, because hypertrophic synovium may obscure visualization. Adequate inflow decreases the possibility of thermal damage to cartilage and soft tissue structures when using a radiofrequency device. Compared with alternative imaging modalities, arthroscopy provides more precise information regarding the status of the articular cartilage, and this may aid in planning future procedures.[20] Reports of synovectomy have shown good short-term results, although the literature does not report maintenance of the short-term benefits over the long-term.[14,20] Therefore, it seems that the usefulness of MCP arthroscopy for inflammatory arthropathy is to aid in diagnosis through synovial biopsy, as well as for staging of articular cartilage involvement. A short-term palliative benefit has also been shown with synovectomy (**Figs. 8** and **9**).

Degenerative arthritis/cartilage lesions

Isolated cartilage lesions and early degenerative arthritis can be assessed, staged, and treated arthroscopically. Debridement of loose cartilage and chondroplasty has been reported in the literature. Good intermediate-term results have been noted with chondroplasty for isolated full-thickness cartilage lesions (**Figs. 10** and **11**).[10]

However, there are no established guidelines outlining a treatment algorithm for degenerative arthritis.

Removal of loose bodies

Similar to larger joints, loose body removal can be performed on the MCP joints of the digits and the thumb (**Figs. 12** and **13**). The unicompartmental nature of the joint facilitates localization and removal of loose bodies. The minimally invasive approach is preferable, because it permits rapid return to activity by obviating incision in the extensor expansion and capsulotomy.

Intra-articular fractures

Fractures involving the articular surfaces and supporting subchondral bone of the MCP joint can be assessed, and treated with an arthroscopically assisted approach (**Figs. 14–16**). K-wires may be used as joysticks to assist reduction, and can also be used for definitive fixation. Alternatively, small conventional screws or headless screws

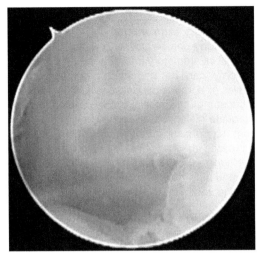

Fig. 8. MCP: inflammatory arthropathy preoperatively.

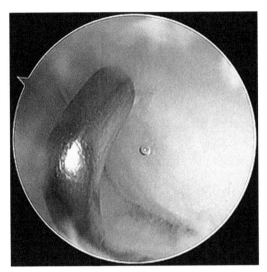

Fig. 10. MCP: after traumatic cartilage lesion.

can be used based on surgeon preference and fracture pattern.

Collateral ligament repair

Ligament injuries in the digits and thumb can be treated with arthroscopically assisted repair. In the thumb, reduction of Stener lesions and joint stabilization has been reported for the treatment of acute unstable UCL injuries (**Figs. 17** and **18**).[17]

The thumb MCP joint is ideally suited for arthroscopically assisted arthrodesis. For individuals with widespread cartilage loss, or with gross instability, fusion may be indicated. Arthroscopic preparation of the joint surfaces and percutaneous cannulated screw fixation are a minimally invasive alternative to open arthrodesis.

The MCP joint of the thumb is ideally suited for arthroscopically assisted fusion. However,

maintenance of mobility is of paramount importance for the MCP joints of the digits. Arthroscopically assisted joint resurfacing may be of benefit for the digits. Arthroscopic evaluation and assistance in preparation of the joint surface for osteocartilagenous transplant can be performed and may play an expanded role in the treatment of isolated articular cartilage defects. In vitro analysis of arthroscopically assisted joint surface preparation for insertion of synthetic or denatured allograft material is under way; this technique may hold great promise for the future and further study, including in vivo analysis, is warranted.

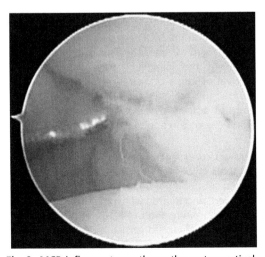

Fig. 9. MCP: inflammatory arthropathy postoperatively.

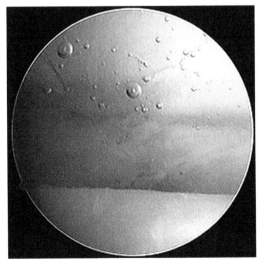

Fig. 11. MCP: after traumatic cartilage lesion after chondroplasty.

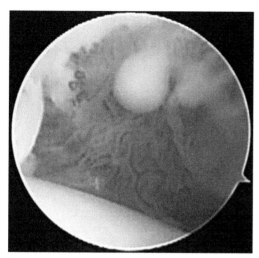

Fig. 12. MCP: loose body.

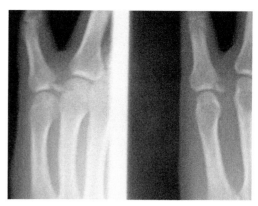

Fig. 14. MCP: articular fracture.

Summary of MCP Joint Arthroscopy

The MCP joint is ideally suited for arthroscopic evaluation and treatment. Nonetheless, the paucity of information in the literature suggests that operative arthroscopy of the MCP joints remains less commonly performed when compared with other joints in the upper extremity such as the wrist, elbow, and shoulder. Further awareness and study will likely expand the application of arthroscopy to surgery to the MCP joints.

PT ARTHROSCOPY

Pisotriquetral arthroscopy is a novel, yet seldom indicated procedure that makes the gee-whiz list. It is indicated for persistent, painful PT joint arthrosis unresponsive to conservative care. PT arthroscopy is also useful for synovectomy, irrigation debridement of septic joints, arthrodesis, or loose body removal.[23]

The hand is suspended by finger-trap traction for convenience of positioning. Two portals are localized with 18-gauge needles under fluoroscopy (**Fig. 19**). Both are placed ulnar to the PT joint, one proximal and one distal. Access to the PT joint can be obtained via the 6R wrist portal in some patients.[24] From the 6R portal, the arthroscope is directed ulnarly, volarly, and distally. Access depends on the presence or absence of a membrane separating the PT joint from the wrist joint. Membrane, if present, can be debrided for entry into the PT joint. However, we prefer direct entry from the ulnar portals.

Incisions are made through the skin. A small, blunt hemostat is used to gain entrance into the PT joint. A 1.9-mm, 30° arthroscope and a 2-mm

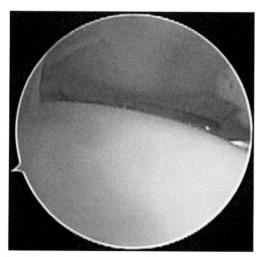

Fig. 13. MCP: after removal of loose body.

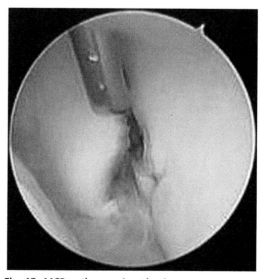

Fig. 15. MCP: arthroscopic reduction.

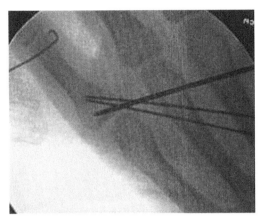

Fig. 16. MCP: arthroscopically assisted percutaneous reduction.

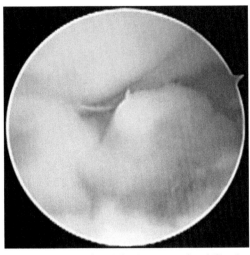

Fig. 18. MCP: UCL after debridement and mobilization.

shaver are used to perform synovectomy and clear the joint of debris. A 2-mm bur is used to remove 2 mm of bone from the pisiform and triquetrum (Fig. 20). The portals are closed with Steri-Strips after the procedure. A short-arm splint is used for 1 week.

Illustrative Case

A 57-year-old woman presented with a several-year history of ulnar-sided wrist/hand pain. She had pain with palpation over the PT joint. PT arthritis was noted on the plane film, and a bone scan showed uptake at the PT joint. She had immediate relief of pain with an injection of local anesthetic into the PT joint under fluoroscopic control. A cortisone injection of the PT joint gave only temporary relief of pain.

A diagnostic injection test has to be interpreted with some caution and in context with other findings of the workup because many patients do not have a membrane separating the PT joint from the radiocarpal joint.[24] Therefore, a local anesthetic injection into the PT joint may anesthetize and therefore eliminate pain from adjacent areas of the wrist.

Full-thickness, widespread cartilage loss was noted at the time of arthroscopy (Fig. 21). Arthroscopic resection arthroplasty of PT joint was performed. Two years after arthroscopic resection arthroplasty, she remained essentially pain free.

PIP ARTHROSCOPY

Arthroscopy of the PIP joint has limited usefulness. The indication for arthroscopy of the PIP joint

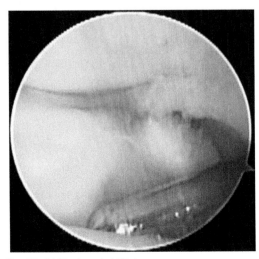

Fig. 17. MCP: chronic UCL tear.

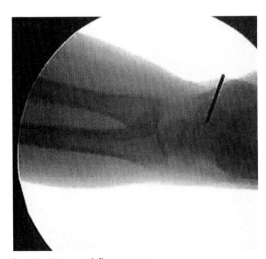

Fig. 19. PT: portal fluoroscopy.

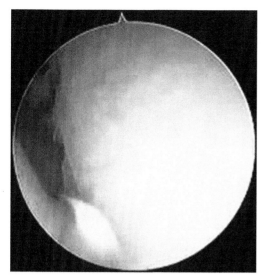

Fig. 20. PT: bur removal of 2 mm of pisiform and triquetrum.

includes synovectomy, irrigation debridement of a septic joint, loose body removal, or diagnostic/staging purposes.[25]

Contraindications include an active cellulitis or severe scarring or contracture of the dorsal tissue secondary to injury or burn.

The authors prefer the use of portals between the lateral bands and collateral ligaments. Portals between the central slip and the lateral bands have also been described.[26]

The digit can be positioned vertically with finger-trap traction or horizontally with manual traction. Because the PIP is a tight bicondylar joint, access to the volar aspect of the joint is limited. Therefore, horizontal positioning allows for joint flexion

and improved access. General or regional anesthesia may be used with either brachial or digital tourniquet.

The joint is distended with saline, and a 3-mm to 4-mm incision is made over the desired portals. Portals can be localized with an 18-gauge needle and fluoroscopy. Blunt spreading with small hemostat allows access into the joint. A tapered blunt trocar is used, and flow is provided through the cannula. The authors use a 1.9-mm, 30° arthroscope (**Fig. 22**). Synovectomy is performed with a 2-mm shaver (**Fig. 23**). Portals are closed with Steri-Strips after the procedure. Early motion is encouraged after synovectomy.

FOURTH AND FIFTH CMC ARTHROSCOPY

The fourth and fifth CMC joints are amenable to arthroscopic evaluation. Usefulness and indications have not been established.

The hand is suspended by finger traps on the fourth and fifth digits with 4.5 kg (10 pounds) of traction. An ulnar portal is localized with an 18-gauge needle and fluoroscopy. The fifth CMC joint is easily viewed arthroscopically through a direct ulnar portal. A dorsal portal is localized with an 18-gauge needle under fluoroscopy (**Fig. 24**). This portal is used for a working portal. A 2-mm shaver is used for synovectomy.

The author uses a 1.9-mm, 30° arthroscope. With the arthroscope in the ulnar portal, the arthroscope can then be transitioned to view across the fifth CMC and into the fourth CMC.

DIP

Arthrodesis of the DIP joint of the fingers or interphalangeal joint of the thumb is an effective surgical treatment of painful arthrosis. The headless screw has been shown to be a safe and effective alternative for fixation with open arthrodesis

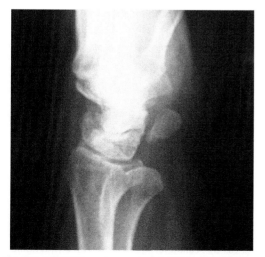

Fig. 21. PT: cartilage loss noted during arthroscopy.

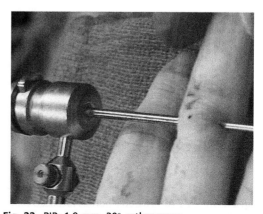

Fig. 22. PIP: 1.9-mm, 30° arthroscope.

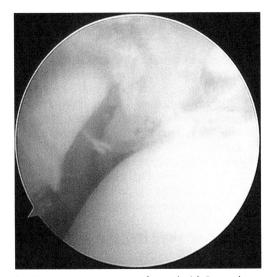

Fig. 23. PIP: synovectomy performed with 2-mm shaver.

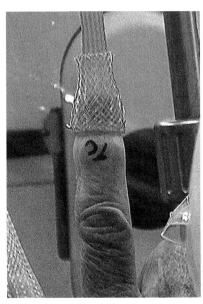

Fig. 25. DIP: digit suspended in finger-trap traction.

techniques.[27–29] Arthroscopic arthrodesis of the DIP joint of the fingers or interphalangeal joint of the thumb is indicated for pain, deformity, or instability. Common causes include degenerative or posttraumatic arthritis, chronic mallet finger, and chronic flexor digitorum profundus injury. This is a technically challenging procedure and should be reserved for only very experienced arthroscopists. The learning curve is steep and the risk of scope damage is high. Contraindications include active infection, bony geometry too small to allow for safe placement of headless screws, and lack

of equipment or experience to safely perform procedure.

Surgical Technique

The digit is suspended with finger-trap traction (**Fig. 25**). This traction is accomplished by turning a standard disposable finger trap inside out to double the wall. It is then placed over the distal phalanx and secured with a transverse 0.35 K-wire through the distal phalanx. The procedure can be performed with a digital or brachial tourniquet. General or regional anesthesia can be used. Traction of 2.3 to 4.5 kg (5–10 pounds) is applied.

Eighteen-gauge needles are used to localize the medial and lateral joint lines under fluoroscopy. Longitudinal incisions are placed over the medial and lateral sides of the joint, 5 to 6 mm long.

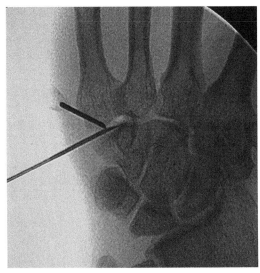

Fig. 24. 5th CMC Arthroscopic portals localized under fluroscopy.

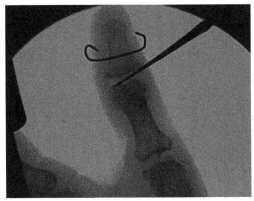

Fig. 26. DIP: collateral ligaments released with number 69 Beaver blade.

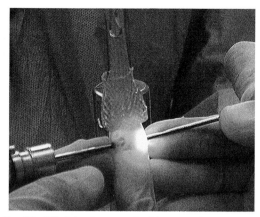

Fig. 27. DIP: joint is opened with Freer elevator.

The collateral ligaments are released with a number 69 Beaver blade. The joint is opened enough to create a working space with a Freer elevator (**Fig. 26**). A 1.9-mm arthroscope is inserted in 1 side of the joint, and a 2.5-mm shaver is inserted in the opposite side of the joint (**Fig. 27**). The joint is cleared of debris. The scope and shaver are then switched, and the opposite side of the joint is cleared of debris, allowing for visualization of both sides of the joint.

Next a 2-mm hooded bur is brought into the joint and 1 to 2 mm of bone is removed from the proximal and distal sides of the joint (**Fig. 28**). Only one-half of the medial and lateral dimensions of the joints are burred to minimize arthroscope damage. The scope and the bur are then switched, and the other side of the joint is burred down to bleeding subchondral bone. Care must be taken not to damage the scope because the working space is limited. Dorsal osteophytes can be removed by palpating the osteophyte under the dorsal capsule and carefully working the bur along the dorsal margin of the joint. The amount of bone resection is assessed visually through the scope and also with the aid of fluoroscopy. If dorsal osteophytes are large, a small flat rasp can be placed dorsally under the extensor tendon for removal.

After resection of the joint the finger trap and transverse fixation wire are removed. A longitudinal guide wire is then placed in the central axis under fluoroscopic control. A cannulated drill is used to drill across the DIP joint followed by placement of the screw (**Fig. 29**).

The authors prefer the mini Acutrak screw because it is small enough to minimize the chance of nail bed damage. The guidewire is then removed. Portals are closed with Steri-Strips. A bulky dressing is applied with a splint for 7 to 10 days. A removable splint is then used for protection as needed, based on patient comfort, for 4 weeks. MCP and PIP joints are mobilized immediately after surgery. Clinical healing occurs at about 6 weeks, with radiographic healing at approximately 8 weeks.[30]

Complications

Complications include nonunion, nail bed injury, and infection.[28] One case was complicated by partial thickness skin loss secondary to fluid

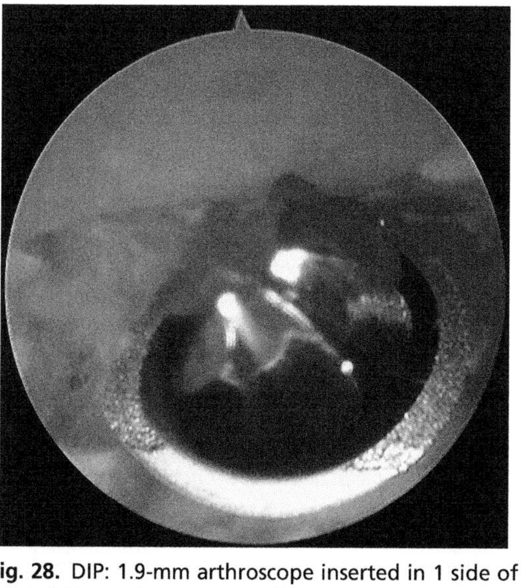

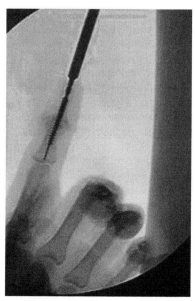

Fig. 28. DIP: 1.9-mm arthroscope inserted in 1 side of joint, 2.5-mm shaver on another.

Fig. 29. DIP: 2-mm hooded bur removes bone from joint.

infiltration.[30] This complication resolved by the second week postoperatively without additional treatment. Medial and lateral approaches place the digital nerves at risk. Care should be taken to avoid injury to these structures.

REFERENCES

1. Eaton RG, Glickel SZ. Trapeziometacarpal osteoarthritis. Staging as a rationale for treatment. Hand Clin 1987;3:455–71.
2. Badia A. Trapeziometacarpal arthroscopy: a classification and treatment algorithm. Hand Clinics 2006; 22(2):153–63.
3. Wilson J. Osteotomy of the first metacarpal in the treatment of arthritis of the carpometacarpal joint of the thumb. Brit J Surg 1973;60:854–8.
4. Badia A, Khachandani P. Treatment of early basal joint arthritis using a combined arthroscopic debridement and metacarpal osteotomy. Tech Hand Up Extrem Surg 2007;11(2):168–73.
5. Tomaino MM. Treatment of Eaton stage I trapeziometacarpal disease. Ligament reconstruction or thumb metacarpal extension osteotomy? Hand Clin 2001; 17:197–205.
6. Cobb T, Sterbank P, Lemke J. Arthroscopic resection arthroplasty for treatment of combined carpometacarpal and scaphotrapeziotrapezoid (pantrapezial) arthritis. J Hand Surg 2011;36(3):413–9.
7. Berner SH. Metacarpophalangeal arthroscopy: techniques and applications. Metacarpophalangeal joint arthroscopy-techniques and applications. Tech Hand Up Extrem Surg 2008;12(4):208–15.
8. Chen YC. Arthroscopy of the wrist and finger joints. Orthop Clin North Am 1979;10:723–33.
9. Rozmaryn L, Wei N. Metacarpophalangeal arthroscopy. Arthroscopy 1999;15(3):333–7.
10. Vaupel G, Andrews J. Diagnostic and operative arthroscopy of the thumb metacarpophalangeal joint: a case report. Am J Sports Med 1985;13(2):139–41.
11. Gaspar L, Szekanecz Z, Dezso B, et al. Technique of synovial biopsy of the metacarpophalangeal joint using the needle athroscope. Knee Surg Sports Traumatol Arthrosc 2003;11:50–2.
12. Kraan M, Reece R, Smeets T, et al. Comparison of synovial tissues from the knee joints and the small joints of rheumatoid arthritis patients: implications for pathogenesis and evaluation of treatment. Arthritis Rheum 2002;46(8):2034–8.
13. Ostendorf B, Dann P, Wedekind F, et al. Miniarthroscopy of the metacarpophalangeal joints in rheumatoid arthritis. Rating of diagnostic value in synovitis staging and efficiency of synovial biopsy. J Rheumatol 1999;26: 1901–8.
14. Wilkes LL. Arthroscopic synovectomy in the rheumatoid metacarpophalangeal joint. J Med Assoc Ga 1987;76:638–9.
15. Ostendorf B, Peters R, Dann P, et al. Magnetic resonance imaging and miniarthroscopy of metacarpophalangeal joints: sensitive detection of morphologic changes in rheumatoid arthritis. Arthritis Rheum 2001;44(11):2492–502.
16. Sekiya I, Kobayashi M, Taneda Y, et al. Arthroscopy of the proximal interphalangeal and metacarpophalangeal joints in rheumatoid hands. Arthroscopy 2002;18(3):292–7.
17. Ryu J, Fagan R. Arthroscopic treatment of acute complete thumb metacarpophalangeal ulnar collateral ligament tears. J Hand Surg Am 1995;20: 1037–42.
18. Slade J III, Gutow A. Arthroscopy of the metacarpophalangeal joint. Hand Clin 1999;15(3):501–26.
19. Declercq G, Schmitgen G, Vestreken J. Athroscopic treatment of metacarpophalangeal arthropathy in haemochromatosis. J Hand Surg 1994; 19(2):212–4.
20. Wei N, Delauter SK, Erlichman MS, et al. Arthroscopic synovectomy of the metacarpophalangeal joint in refractory rheumatoid arthritis: a technique. Arthroscopy 1999;15(3):265–8.
21. Badia A. Arthroscopic reduction and internal fixation of bony gamekeeper's thumb. Tips and techniques. Orthopedics 2006;29(8):675–8.
22. Badia A. Arthroscopy of the trapeziometacarpal and metacarpophalangeal joints. J Hand Surg Am 2007; 32(5):707–24.
23. Katolik LI. Arthroscopic resection, pisotriquetral joint loose body: a case report. J Hand Surg Am 2008; 32(2):2006–9.
24. Aroya AP, Aulshreshtha R, Kakarala GK, et al. Visualization of pisotriquetral joint through standard portals for arthroscopy of the wrist: a clinical and anatomical study. J Bone Joint Surg Br 2007;89(2):202–5.
25. Sekya I, Kobayashi M, Okamoto H, et al. Arthroscopic synovectomy metacarpophalangeal and proximal interphalangeal joint. Tech Hand Up Extrem Surg 2008;12(4):221–5.
26. Thomsen MO, Mielsen MS, Gorgensen U, et al. Arthroscopy of the proximal interphalangeal joints and fingers. J Hand Surg Br 2002;27:253–5.
27. Leibovic SJ. Instructional course lecture. Arthrodesis of the interphalangeal joints with headless compression screws. J Hand Surg Am 2007;32(7):1113–9.
28. Brutus JP, Palmer AK, Mosher JF, et al. Use of a headless compression screw for distal interphalangeal joint arthrodesis in digits: clinical outcome and review of complications. J Hand Surg Am 2006;31(1):85–9.
29. Tuttle HG, Olvey SP, Stern P. Tendon avulsion injuries of the distal phalanx. Clin Orthop Relat 2006;445: 157–68.
30. Cobb TK. Arthroscopic distal interphalangeal joint arthrodesis. Tech Hand Up Extrem Surg 2008; 12(4):266–9.

Arthroscopic Synovectomy of the Wrist

Lars Adolfsson, MD

KEYWORDS

- Arthroscopic synovectomy • Wrist arthritis
- Rheumatoid arthritis • Synovitis

The possibility of arthroscopic synovectomy of the wrist was probably first mentioned by Roth and Poehling[1] in 1990. This finding was during a period when the technique of wrist arthroscopy was evolving, following the pioneering work by Whipple and colleagues[2] a few years earlier. Early and mid-term results of synovectomy in rheumatoid arthritis (RA) were then reported shortly thereafter by this author,[3,4] and equally beneficial outcomes were later presented by Tünnerhoff and Haussmann[5] in 2002 and also by Park and colleagues[6] in 2003. There are still few studies presenting results after this procedure and still no comparative studies using control groups. To date, results from little more than 100 procedures can be found in the literature. The published short- and intermediate-term results, however, suggest that in RA, arthroscopic wrist synovectomy can provide a marked reduction of pain and an improved function.[3,4,6–8] The technique has also been used for other diagnoses causing wrist arthritis, but very few results have been reported and the indications remain to be defined.

The rationale of a surgical synovectomy is to excise inflamed synovium and thereby remove as much effusion and inflammatory substrate as possible. The excised synovium is replaced by a new lining of cells that resembles normal synovial membrane but with some different functions.[9,10] It has been found that if the procedure is performed at an early stage of the disease, before the joint has been affected by major irreversible changes, symptoms may be markedly reduced for a considerable time.[4,11–16] In most cases, however, the effect seems not to be permanent, but whether this is a true recurrence or overgrowth from residuals after an incomplete excision is unknown. How rapid the synovitis will recur and how intense the inflammatory reaction will be probably depend on the activity of the underlying arthritic disease. Some have claimed that synovectomy in RA can have a good effect of considerable duration and perhaps even halt further joint deterioration.[11,12,14–18] This claim has, however, been based on anecdotal reports and has not been substantiated in larger materials.[17,19,20] Two multi-center studies of large series of synovectomies from different joints could not document any long-lasting effect on radiographic appearance.[19,20] At present, there seems to be a general agreement that in systemic arthritic diseases, the beneficial effect is local and transitory.[21] There are, however, conditions, such as postinfectious monoarthritis, in which the effect seems to be permanent and, in some cases, perhaps even curative.

INDICATIONS

Improved medication has dramatically improved the treatment of many arthritic diseases during the past decades, and the need for surgical synovectomy has been reduced. Arthroscopic synovectomy may be indicated in any kind of disease that leads to a long-standing synovitis of the wrist and when other treatment modalities do not provide satisfactorily symptom reduction or may be contraindicated. In a more acute situation, arthroscopic synovectomy may also be considered in the treatment of bacterial arthritis. If the synovitis is a part of a chronic arthritic condition,

Department of Orthopaedic Surgery, Linköping University Hospital, Linköping 58185, Sweden
E-mail address: Lars.Adolfsson@lio.se

Hand Clin 27 (2011) 395–399
doi:10.1016/j.hcl.2011.06.001
0749-0712/11/$ – see front matter © 2011 Elsevier Inc. All rights reserved.

it is recommended that the decision of an arthroscopic synovectomy is taken in agreement with a rheumatologist.

The main indication for arthroscopic synovectomy remains to be in patients with RA in whom pharmacologic treatment has not been tolerated or sufficiently effective to reduce joint synovitis. In general, all patients who are considered for surgery should at least once have tried intra-articular steroid injections and have had persistent joint synovitis for more than 6 months. The patient typically presents with tender elastic swelling dorsally over the radiocarpal and midcarpal joints. Palpable synovitis around the distal ulna and sixth extensor tendon compartment is a frequent accompanying finding. In the event of associated extensor tendon synovitis, a careful clinical examination is essential to differentiate these locations because both might have to be addressed. If an open simultaneous procedure is indicated, the decision of arthroscopic synovectomy is guided by the desired postoperative regime.

Extensive open wrist surgery is normally avoided in connection with arthroscopic synovectomy, but minor procedures that allow early mobilization are not discouraged.[7]

Marked arthritic changes on plain radiographs, severity of grade III or more according to the staging system by Larsen, Dale, Eek (LDE index),[22] have been found to be associated with disappointing results, and arthroscopic synovectomy is presently only recommended for patients with radiographic changes of grade 0 to II on the LDE index.[4,7] The index is a radiographic classification in 6 stages describing the severity of arthritic changes, where 0 means no changes and grade II, early changes with slight joint space narrowing and possible periarticular minor erosions. Grade III represents medium destructive abnormality with definite erosions and joint space narrowing, whereas grades IV and V encompass increasingly severe forms of arthritic joint destruction. Patients with juvenile chronic arthritis (JCA) have been treated similarly based on findings in studies on open synovectomy for this diagnosis, indicating that the results do not differ from those in adult RA.[16,23]

Of the other connective tissue diseases associated with chronic wrist synovitis, systemic lupus erythematosus (SLE) has most frequently been treated with arthroscopic synovectomy. The experiences have been similar to the outcome after operation in patients with RA.[7]

In patients with long-standing symptoms because of postinfectious monoarthritis, arthroscopic synovectomy has been found beneficial.[7] The results have been stable for many years, and, unlike in RA, there has been no sign of the synovitis to recur and no sign of radiographic deterioration has been observed.

Treatment of septic arthritis of the wrist has been advocated, and results have been encouraging in the relatively few reported cases.[7,24,25] Sammer and Shin[26] found arthroscopic treatment effective with fewer reoperations and shorter hospital stay than after open surgery. The procedure has been described to include biopsy for cultures, repeat lavage, and resection of inflamed synovium in the radiocarpal joint and midcarpal space.[7,26]

Synovectomy is often an integral part of the procedures for treating conditions of degenerative nature amenable for arthroscopic surgery, such as wafer resection for ulnar impaction syndrome, debridement in scaphotrapeziotrapezoid (STT) osteoarthritis, radial styloidectomy for styloid impaction on the scaphoid, and triangular fibrocartilage complex (TFCC) resections for degenerative changes.

Radial plica is a condition in which a hypertrophic synovial fold over the radial styloid may impinge between the scaphoid and the styloid, producing localized pain and snapping.[3] This condition has successfully been treated with resection of the fibrotic and hypertrophic synovium.

Synovitis may occur in connection with arthrofibrosis following trauma or surgery to the wrist. In these cases, synovectomy; release of adhesions; and, occasionally, capsular release can significantly reduce symptoms and improve joint mobility.[7,27,28]

CONTRAINDICATIONS

Arthroscopic synovectomy has been tried in psoriatic arthropathy, but the results have been reported to be unpredictable at best, and the procedure is not recommended in this disease.[7] Patients with an unstable soft tissue envelope are also not suitable candidates. Simultaneous procedures that require postoperative immobilization are not an absolute contraindication, but the advantageous effect of immediate training is obviously lost. Other relative contraindications include patients with other severe arthritic manifestations in the same arm who may not be able to manage the position normally used for wrist arthroscopy and patients with previous arthroplasties in the finger joints.

TECHNIQUE

Standard techniques and instrumentation for wrist arthroscopy is used, adhering closely to the previously published detailed technical descriptions.[2,3,6–8,29–33] The hand is suspended in a conventional traction device with Chinese finger traps. In patients with RA, care is taken to minimize the amount of traction and to distribute the traction to all fingers because many patients have increased laxity of the wrist and finger joint ligaments and frail skin. Continuous irrigation using an automatic pressure-regulated pump is preferred, but passive infusion from an elevated bag of saline solution through a separate inflow cannula is possible.

The standard 3–4 and 6R portals are normally used for surgery in the radiocarpal joint. Using the same skin incisions, midcarpal, radial, and ulnar portals are established. Depending on the location of intra-articular pathologies, the 6U, distal radioulnar joint (DRUJ), and STT portals have been used. Volar portals have so far not been found necessary.

A 2.9-mm shaver blade is preferred, but occasionally 2-mm blades can be used in narrow parts of the joints. Thermocoagulation has been advocated because the small-diameter probes facilitate access and the procedure is more rapid. Potentially adverse effects of heat development around the probes have become a concern because the limited irrigation that can be achieved through the small arthroscopic sheath may not provide sufficient cooling. Serious complications have been reported,[34] and, besides extreme caution in handling, additional irrigation through a separate inflow cannula may be recommendable.

In arthritis caused by RA or other connective tissue diseases, the synovitis is usually typically distributed in areas of the joint that are most mobile and where there is abundance of joint capsule. In the radiocarpal joint, most are found in the radial and ulnar recesses, on the dorsal capsule, and adjacent to the radioscapholunate ligament of Testut. In the midcarpal space, most of the synovitis can be found in the STT joint, on the dorsoulnar capsule, and volarly under the capitohamate joint. The author believes that the intra-articular distribution of synovitis is a result of how much the respective parts of the joint can move. Consequently, there are more capsular tissues and folds in these areas.

The DRUJ is also often affected, frequently in conjunction with a degenerative TFCC lesion and increased laxity of the DRUJ capsule. This condition facilitates synovectomy, which can be performed both through a central defect in the horizontal part of the TFCC or via separate DRUJ portals.

Postoperatively, a light bandage is applied and kept for 12 to 14 days at which time the arthroscopy portals are usually healed. Immediate movement exercises are begun after the surgery, and unrestricted load bearing is allowed after the wounds are healed.

RESULTS

Arthroscopic synovectomy in rheumatoid wrists with no or mild radiographic changes has been reported to reduce pain and improve function, range of motion, and grip strength in short- and intermediate-term follow-ups.[3,4,6–8,29] Although the design of the published studies does not allow definite conclusions on the efficacy of the procedure, the collected data suggest that a relatively long period of increased comfort can be expected in patients with RA. In a recent follow-up, 21 patients were identified having had an arthroscopic synovectomy between 1991 and 1994 (Adolfsson L, MD, and Kalén A, MD, unpublished data, 2010). Eighteen patients who were alive could be localized and were interviewed. Fourteen accepted a visit for clinical examination and control radiographs. Of these, 11 had been diagnosed with RA, 1 with SLE, and 2 with postinfectious monoarthritis. In addition, the authors examined 2 patients who had been operated 12 and 15 years earlier, respectively, because of postinfectious arthritis.

It was found that only 1 patient had undergone additional surgery in the same wrist. Six regarded themselves as free from wrist symptoms; 9 had mild symptoms, such as slight weakness and sensation of instability, whereas 5 had moderate pain and stiffness. All patients with postinfectious arthritis denied any discomfort from the wrist, and no radiographic abnormalities were found. Two of the patients diagnosed with RA still had no radiological signs of arthritic changes, but, with the remaining 9, there were signs of deterioration. In general, the accentuated changes corresponded to one stage in the LDE index. The radiographic changes did, however, not necessarily correlate with increased symptoms. Most patients with RA had at some point during the follow-up period changed their medication and at least 6 had tried, or were on, immunosuppressive treatment, making interpretation of the results even more difficult.

In posttraumatic synovitis and arthrofibrosis, the synovectomy and removal of intra-articular adhesions usually resulted in improvements within a few weeks after the operations and the initial gains in range of motion seem to remain stable.[27]

Complications after wrist arthroscopy have been reported to be rare, and, in the experience of arthroscopic synovectomy, the only recorded complication that has required additional treatment was a synovial fistula that did not heal despite immobilization and consequently was excised 5 weeks after the initial operation.[7]

SUMMARY

Arthroscopic synovectomy is safe and reliable, with mild postoperative morbidity. In most cases, this technique is performed as an outpatient procedure. In RA and most likely also in JCA, SLE, and postinfectious monoarthritis, a relatively long period of increased comfort and improved function can be anticipated. The procedure may be considered in posttraumatic cases with joint contracture and as an adjunct to other measures for certain osteoarthritic disorders. In septic arthritis with insufficient clinical improvement after systemic antibiotics and lavage, arthroscopic synovectomy seems advantageous.

It should, however, be borne in mind that the reported results must be viewed in relation to the level of activity of each patient. Many patients who are affected by a connective tissue disease have its effects in many locations and may consequently have relatively low functional demands. Therefore, the results must be interpreted with caution, and generalizations should be minimized. Even though some patients rate their wrist as being free of symptoms, an objective examination will, in most cases, reveal some dysfunction and not an entirely normal wrist. For most patients with arthritic disease, the arthroscopic synovectomy can provide locally reduced symptoms but rarely a normal wrist.

REFERENCES

1. Roth JH, Poehling GG. Arthroscopic "-ectomy" surgery of the wrist. Arthroscopy 1990;6:141–7.
2. Whipple TL, Marotta JJ, Powell JH. Techniques of wrist arthroscopy. Arthroscopy 1986;2:244–52.
3. Adolfsson L, Nylander G. Arthroscopic synovectomy of the rheumatoid wrist. J Hand Surg 1993;18B: 92–6.
4. Adolfsson L, Frisén M. Arthroscopic synovectomy of the rheumatoid wrist—a 3.8 year follow-up. J Hand Surg 1997;22B:711–3.
5. Tünnerhoff HG, Haussmann P. Results of arthroscopic synovialectomy of the wrist. Handchir Mikrochir Plast Chir 2002;34(3):158–67 [in German].
6. Park MJ, Ahn JH, Kang JS. Arthroscopic synovectomy of the wrist in rheumatoid arthritis. J Bone Joint Surg Br 2003;85:1011–5.
7. Adolfsson L. Arthroscopic synovectomy in wrist arthritis. Hand Clin 2005;21:527–30.
8. Wei N, Delauter SK, Beard S, et al. Office-based arthroscopic synovectomy of the wrist in rheumatoid arthritis. Arthroscopy 2001;17:884–7.
9. Goldie I, Wellisch M. The presence of nerves in original and regenerated synovial tissue in patients synovectomised for rheumatoid arthritis. Acta Orthop Scand 1969;40:143–52.
10. Mitchell N, Shepard N. The effect of synovectomy on synovium and cartilage in early rheumatoid arthritis. Clin Orthop 1972;889:178–96.
11. Aschan W, Moberg E. A long-term study on the effect of early synovectomy in rheumatoid arthritis. Bull Hosp Jt Dis Orthop Inst 1984;44:106–21.
12. Ishikawa H, Ohno O, Hirohata K. Long-term results of synovectomy in rheumatoid patients. J Bone Joint Surg Am 1986;68:198–205.
13. Jensen CM, Poulsen S, Östergren M, et al. Early and late synovectomy of the knee in rheumatoid arthritis. Scand J Rheumatol 1991;20:127–31.
14. Matsui N, Taneda Y, Ohta H, et al. Arthroscopic versus open synovectomy in the rheumatoid knee. Int Orthop 1989;13:17–20.
15. Pahle JA, Kvarnes L. Shoulder synovectomy. Ann Chir Gynaecol Suppl 1985;74(Suppl 198):37–9.
16. Vahvanen V, Pätiälä H. Synovectomy of the wrist in rheumatoid arthritis and related diseases. Arch Orthop Trauma Surg 1984;102:230–7.
17. Böhler N, Lack N, Schwägerl W, et al. Late results of synovectomy of wrist, MP and PIP joints: multicenter study. Clin Rheumatol 1985;4:23–5.
18. Ferlic DC, Clayton ML. Synovectomy of the hand and wrist. Ann Chir Gynaecol Suppl 1985;74(Suppl 198): 26–30.
19. Arthritis Foundation Committee on Evaluation of Synovectomy: multi-center evaluation of synovectomy in the treatment of rheumatoid arthritis: report of results at the end of three years. Arthritis Rheum 1977;20: 765–71.
20. Arthritis and Rheumatism Council and British Orthopaedic Association: controlled trial of synovectomy of knee and metacarpophalangeal joints in rheumatoid arthritis. Ann Rheum Dis 1976;35: 437–42.
21. Feldon P, Terrono AL, Nalebuff EA, et al. Rheumatoid arthritis and other connective tissue diseases. In: Green DP, Hotchkiss RN, Pederson WC, editors. Green's operative hand surgery. Philadelphia: Churchill Livingstone; 1999. p. 1651–739.
22. Larsen A, Dale K, Eek M. Radiographic evaluation of rheumatoid arthritis and related conditions by standard reference films. Acta Radiol Diagn (Stockh) 1977;18:481–91.
23. Hanff G, Sollerman C, Elborgh R, et al. Wrist synovectomy in rheumatoid arthritis. Scand J Rheumatol 1990;19:280–4, 9.
24. Bain GI, Roth JH. The role of arthroscopy in arthritis. Hand Clin 1995;11:51–8.
25. Parisien JS, Shaffer B. Arthroscopic management of pyarthrosis. Clin Orthop 1992;275:243–7.
26. Sammer DM, Shin AY. Comparison of arthroscopic and open treatment of septic arthritis of the wrist. J Bone Joint Surg Am 2009;91:1387–93.

27. Luchetti R, Atzei A, Fairplay T. Arthroscopic wrist ar-
    throlysis after wrist fracture. Arthroscopy 2007;23(3):
    255–60.
28. Osterman AL. Wrist arthroscopy: operative proce-
    dures. In: Green DP, Hotchkiss RN, Pederson WC,
    editors. Green's operative hand surgery. Philadel-
    phia: Churchill Livingstone; 1999. p. 207–22.
29. Adolfsson L. Open vs. arthroscopic synovectomy of
    the wrist. In: Trail I, Hayton M, editors. Surgery of the
    rheumatoid hand and wrist, international congress
    series 1295. Amsterdam: Elsevier; 2006. p. 56–62.
30. Bain GI, Richards RS, Roth JM. Arthroscopy of the
    wrist: introduction and indications. In: McGinty JB,

Caspari RB, Jackson RW, et al, editors. Operative
arthroscopy. Philadelphia: Lippincott-Raven; 1996.
p. 897–904.
31. Botte MJ, Cooney WP, Linscheid RL. Arthroscopy of
    the wrist: anatomy and technique. J Hand Surg
    1989;14A:313–6.
32. Roth JH. Hand instrumentation for small joint arthro-
    scopy. Arthroscopy 1988;4:126–8.
33. Whipple TL. Powered instruments for wrist arthros-
    copy. Arthroscopy 1988;4:290–4.
34. Pell RF IV, Uhl RL. Complications of thermal ablation
    in wrist arthroscopy. Arthroscopy 2004;20(Suppl 2):
    84–6.

Index

Hand Clin 27 (2011) 401–403
doi:10.1016/S0749-0712(11)00056-4
0749-0712/11/$ – see front matter © 2011 Elsevier Inc. All rights reserved.

Moving?

Make sure your subscription moves with you!

To notify us of your new address, find your **Clinics Account Number** (located on your mailing label above your name), and contact customer service at:

Email: journalscustomerservice-usa@elsevier.com

800-654-2452 (subscribers in the U.S. & Canada)
314-447-8871 (subscribers outside of the U.S. & Canada)

Fax number: 314-447-8029

Elsevier Health Sciences Division
Subscription Customer Service
3251 Riverport Lane
Maryland Heights, MO 63043

*To ensure uninterrupted delivery of your subscription, please notify us at least 4 weeks in advance of move.

Printed and bound by CPI Group (UK) Ltd, Croydon, CR0 4YY

03/10/2024

01040357-0007